T0419355

GLOBAL HIV/AIDS THREAT AND THE U.S. RESPONSE

PUBLIC HEALTH IN THE 21ST CENTURY

Additional books in this series can be found on Nova's website
under the Series tab.

Additional E-books in this series can be found on Nova's website
under the E-books tab.

GLOBAL HIV/AIDS THREAT AND THE U.S. RESPONSE

DAVID R. CARMODY

EDITOR

Nova Science Publishers, Inc.

New York

For permission to use material from this book please contact us:
Telephone 631-231-7269; Fax 631-231-8175
Web Site: http://www.novapublishers.com

NOTICE TO THE READER

The Publisher has taken reasonable care in the preparation of this book, but makes no expressed or implied warranty of any kind and assumes no responsibility for any errors or omissions. No liability is assumed for incidental or consequential damages in connection with or arising out of information contained in this book. The Publisher shall not be liable for any special, consequential, or exemplary damages resulting, in whole or in part, from the readers' use of, or reliance upon, this material. Any parts of this book based on government reports are so indicated and copyright is claimed for those parts to the extent applicable to compilations of such works.

Independent verification should be sought for any data, advice or recommendations contained in this book. In addition, no responsibility is assumed by the publisher for any injury and/or damage to persons or property arising from any methods, products, instructions, ideas or otherwise contained in this publication.

This publication is designed to provide accurate and authoritative information with regard to the subject matter covered herein. It is sold with the clear understanding that the Publisher is not engaged in rendering legal or any other professional services. If legal or any other expert assistance is required, the services of a competent person should be sought. FROM A DECLARATION OF PARTICIPANTS JOINTLY ADOPTED BY A COMMITTEE OF THE AMERICAN BAR ASSOCIATION AND A COMMITTEE OF PUBLISHERS.

Additional color graphics may be available in the e-book version of this book.

Library of Congress Cataloging-in-Publication Data

Global HIV/AIDS threat and the U.S. response / editor, David R. Carmody.
    p. ; cm.
  Includes bibliographical references and index.
  ISBN 978-1-61324-568-2 (hardcover)
  1. HIV infections. 2. AIDS (Disease) 3. Medical policy--United States--International Cooperation. I. Carmody, David R.
  [DNLM: 1. HIV Infections--United States. 2. Acquired Immunodeficiency Syndrome--United States. 3. Health Policy--United States. 4. International Cooperation--United States. WC 503]
  RA643.8.G566 2011
  362.196'9792--dc23
                2011014478

Published by Nova Science Publishers, Inc. + New York

CONTENTS

PREFACE

The human immunodeficiency virus/acquired immune deficiency syndrome (HIV/AIDS) is one of the world's most pressing global health challenges. Since the beginning of the epidemic, more than 60 million people have been infected with HIV, approximately 30 million of whom have died of HIV-related causes. As of 2009, there were 33.3 million people living with the virus, the vast majority of whom live in sub-Saharan Africa. Expanded access to antiretroviral therapy over the past decade, due in large part to U.S. support, has contributed to declines in deaths among people living with HIV. Nonetheless, new infections continue to outpace access to treatment. This book provides information on key components of the HIV/AIDS epidemic and an examination of determining how, and to what extent, the United States should respond to the continued challenge of global HIV/AIDS.

Chapter 1- The human immunodeficiency virus/acquired immune deficiency syndrome (HIV/AIDS) is one of the world's most pressing global health challenges. Since the beginning of the epidemic, more than 60 million people have been infected with HIV, approximately 30 million of whom have died of HIV-related causes. As of 2009, there were 33.3 million people living with the virus, the vast majority of whom live in sub-Saharan Africa. Expanded access to antiretroviral therapy (ART) over the past decade, due in large part to U.S. support, has contributed to declines in deaths among people living with HIV. Nonetheless, new infections continue to outpace access to treatment. The 112th Congress will likely be faced with determining how, and to what extent, the United States should respond to the continued challenge of global HIV/AIDS.

Chapter 2- Launched in 2003 by President George W. Bush, PEPFAR holds a place in history as the largest effort by any nation to combat a single disease. In the first five years of the program, PEPFAR focused on establishing and scaling up prevention, care and treatment programs. It achieved success in expanding access to HIV prevention, care and treatment in low-resource settings. During its first phase, PEPFAR supported the provision of treatment to more than 2 million people, care to more than 10 million people, including more than 4 million orphans and vulnerable children, and prevention of mother-to-child treatment services during nearly 16 million pregnancies.

Chapter 3- Prevention remains the paramount challenge of the HIV epidemic, and preventing new infections represents the only long-term, sustainable way to turn the tide against HIV/AIDS. For any given population, the public health response must strike a balance between prevention opportunities and treatment needs. A successful prevention program requires a combination of mutually reinforcing interventions tailored to the needs of different target populations.

According to the Joint United Nations Programme on HIV/AIDS (UNAIDS), there were approximately 2.7 million new HIV infections in 2008, and 33.4 million people living with HIV.[1] New infections still far outpace the world's ability to add people to treatment. For every two people put on antiretroviral drugs (ARVs), another five become newly infected.[2] In recent years, several low- prevalence countries have had some success in containing their epidemics, concentrated in most-at-risk populations (MARPs). However, only a few high-prevalence countries have significantly reduced HIV prevalence. Increased attention is critical for hyperendemic countries, while simultaneously continuing to respond to countries with both concentrated and generalized epidemics.

Chapter 4- In July 2008, as part of its reauthorization, the U.S. President's Emergency Plan for AIDS Relief (PEPFAR) was encouraged to negotiate framework documents with partner countries. By establishing these partnerships, PEPFAR is promoting and developing a more sustainable approach to the fight against HIV/AIDS at the country level. These Partnership Frameworks are characterized by strengthened country capacity, ownership, and leadership, and represent a substantially new focus for PEPFAR. Partnership Frameworks pave the way for approaches to foreign assistance based upon collaboration on principles that are common to U.S. Government (USG) objectives and partner country plans and activities.

Chapter 5- The President's Emergency Plan for AIDS Relief (PEPFAR), reauthorized at $48 billion for fiscal years 2009 through 2013, supports HIV/AIDS prevention, treatment, and care services overseas. The reauthorizing legislation, as well as other key documents and PEPFAR guidance, endorses the alignment of PEPFAR activities with partner country HIV/AIDS strategies and the promotion of partner country ownership of U.S.-supported HIV/AIDS programs. This report, responding to a legislative directive, (1) examines alignment of PEPFAR programs with partner countries' HIV/AIDS strategies and (2) describes several challenges related to alignment or promotion of country ownership. GAO analyzed PEPFAR planning documents and national strategies for four countries—Cambodia, Malawi, Uganda, and Vietnam—selected to represent factors such as diversity of funding levels and geographic location. GAO also reviewed documents and reports by the U.S. government, research institutions, and international organizations and interviewed PEPFAR officials and other stakeholders in headquarters and the four countries.

Chapter 6- In 2007, UNAIDS reported that 22.5 million people in sub-Saharan Africa were living with HIV/AIDS. This figure represents nearly 68 percent of the total 33.2 million cases worldwide. New infections of HIV among children and adults in Africa in 2007 numbered 2.5 million. Nearly 6 1 percent of HIV infections in this region occur in women, a higher percentage than any part of the world. Approximately 76 percent of the 2.1 million AIDS-related deaths worldwide in 2007 occurred in sub-Saharan Africa, where AIDS is by far the most common cause of mortality, according to the UNAIDS 2007 *Epidemic Update*. In addition, the region is home to an alarming 80 percent of the world's children who have been orphaned or otherwise made vulnerabl e by HIV/AIDS.

Chapter 7- National HIV infection levels in Asia are low compared with those in Africa. HIV prevalence is highest in Southeast Asia, with wide variation in epidemic trends among different countries. Burma and Cambodia show declines in prevalence, but the epidem ic is growing at a particularly high rate in Indonesia (particularly in the Papua Province) and Vietnam. In East Asia, there were almost 20 percent more new HIV infections in 2007 compared with 2001. In South and Southeast Asia, the number of new HIV infection s decreased from 450,000 in 2001 to 340,000 in 2007. Even though prevalence rates may be low, the large populations of many Asian nations mean that large numbers of people have HIV infection. For the Asia region, the latest estimates show that 4 .9 million people were living with HIV in 2007, including 440,000 people who became newly infected in the past year, and that AIDS claimed approximately 300,000 lives in 2007 (UNAIDS, November 2007). In East Asia, approximately 800,000 people were living with HIV, and AIDS claimed 32,000 lives in this subregion in 2007, according to UNAIDS. As of 2005, ap proximately 52,400 people living in Central Asia were HIV positive.

Chapter 8- Most HIV epidemics in the Latin America and Caribbean (LAC) region appear to be stable, although in some Caribbean countries, they appear to be in decline. In 2007, about 69,000 people in LAC countries died of AIDS, and 117,000 were newly infected (UNAIDS, November 2007). The number of people living with HIV/AIDS (PLWHA) in LAC is estimated at 1 .8 million (UNAIDS, November 2007). Two-thirds of PLWHA reside in the four largest countries – Argentina, Brazil, Colombia, and Mexico – although the Caribbean and Central American subregions have higher prevalence rates, with countries such as Haiti and Belize having rates in 2005 as high as 3.8 and 2.5 percent, respectively (see figure below). With its large population, Brazil accounts for about one-third of PLWHA in the region. The epidemics in LAC are being fueled by varying combinations of unsafe sex (both between men and between men and women) and injecting drug use, but it is important to note that HIV/AIDS transmission patterns have moved increasingly from marginalized groups toward the general population·(UNAIDS, December 2006). HIV prevalence among sex workers is relatively high in Central America and the Caribbean, especially in the Dominican Republic, Jamaica, Guyana, Honduras, Guatemala, and El Salvador (UNAIDS, November 2007). Unprotected sex between men is an important factor in Bolivia, Chile, Ecuador, Peru, El Salvador, Guatemala, Honduras, Mexico, Nicaragua, and Panama (UNAIDS, November 2007). Prevalence among men who have sex with men (MSM) may well be underestimated throughout the region because of stigma, the often hidden nature of this behavior, the fact that some MSM also have sex with women, and the small numbers of people engaging in risky behaviors who actually know their status. Between 1986 and 2004, 27 percent of the HIV/AIDS cases in Argentina, Uruguay, Paraguay, and Chile were attributed to injecting drug use, and over the same time period in Brazil, 16 percent of cases were transmitted through injecting drug use (USAID, 2006). However, HIV prevalence in Brazil among injecting drug users (IDUs) is declining in some cities as a result of harm reduction programs, mortality among IDUs, and a change from injecting to inhaling drugs (UNAIDS and WHO, 2006). In Argentina and Uruguay, the epidemics are driven mainly by unprotected heterosexual intercourse (UNAIDS, November 2007).

Chapter 9- Eastern Europe and Central Asia is the only region where HIV prevalence clearly continues to increase, with an estimated 130,000 new infections in 2009 alone. In the same year, 1.4 million adults and children were living with HIV in Eastern Europe and Central Asia. From 2001 to 2008, there was a 66 percent increase in the total number of people living with HIV/AIDS (PLWHA); in comparison, prevalence in sub-Saharan Africa fell from 5.8 percent to 5.2 percent, and prevalence in Southeast Asia stabilized in the same period. Eastern Europe is also the only region where the annual number of HIV-related deaths continues to rise, increasing fourfold from 18,000 in 2001 to 76,000 in 2009.

In: Global HIV/AIDS Threat and the U.S. Response
Editor: David R. Carmody

ISBN: 978-1-61324-568-2
© 2011 Nova Science Publishers, Inc.

Chapter 1

U.S. RESPONSE TO THE GLOBAL THREAT OF HIV/AIDS: BASIC FACTS

Alexandra E. Kendall

SUMMARY

The human immunodeficiency virus/acquired immune deficiency syndrome (HIV/AIDS) is one of the world's most pressing global health challenges. Since the beginning of the epidemic, more than 60 million people have been infected with HIV, approximately 30 million of whom have died of HIV-related causes. As of 2009, there were 33.3 million people living with the virus, the vast majority of whom live in sub-Saharan Africa. Expanded access to antiretroviral therapy (ART) over the past decade, due in large part to U.S. support, has contributed to declines in deaths among people living with HIV. Nonetheless, new infections continue to outpace access to treatment. The 112th Congress will likely be faced with determining how, and to what extent, the United States should respond to the continued challenge of global HIV/AIDS.

The United States has recognized HIV/AIDS as a key foreign policy priority. Congress has passed several pieces of legislation related to global HIV/AIDS prevention, treatment, and care. In particular, in 2003, Congress enacted the U.S. Leadership Against HIV/AIDS, Tuberculosis, and Malaria Act of 2003 (P.L. 108-25), authorizing $15 billion to combat global HIV/AIDS, tuberculosis (TB), and malaria through the President's Emergency Plan for AIDS Relief (PEPFAR), an initiative proposed by the George W. Bush Administration. In 2008, Congress enacted the Tom Lantos and Henry J. Hyde United States Global Leadership Against HIV/AIDS, Tuberculosis, and Malaria Reauthorization Act of 2008 (P.L. 110-293), authorizing $48 billion for HIV/AIDS, TB, and malaria programs from FY2009 through FY2013. From FY2004 through FY2010, the United States spent a total of $26,348 million on bilateral HIV/AIDS programs.

PEPFAR is the largest commitment in history by any nation to combat a single disease and makes up the majority of donor funding for global HIV/AIDS. When PEPFAR was announced, health experts were debating whether the international community had a responsibility to provide ART in developing countries and whether they could be safely administered in such environments. PEPFAR responded to calls from those advocating treatment for the world's poor and demonstrated that ART could be effectively provided in low-resource settings.

PEPFAR is coordinated by the Office of the U.S. Global AIDS Coordinator (OGAC) at the Department of State and is implemented by a range of U.S. agencies that include, among others, the United States Agency for International Development (USAID) and the Centers for Disease Control and Prevention (CDC). The United States also supports several multilateral organizations responding to HIV/AIDS, including the Global Fund to Fight AIDS, Tuberculosis and Malaria (Global Fund) and the United Nations Joint Program on HIV/AIDS (UNAIDS).

Due in part to the global response to HIV/AIDS, progress has been made in combating the epidemic. New HIV infections fell by more than 25% in 33 countries between 2001 and 2009, and AIDS-related deaths have declined significantly. At the same time, major challenges remain in the fight against HIV/AIDS. For example, the number of people in need of treatment has continued to grow, straining available resources. Global health experts have increasingly debated the sustainability of expanded access to HIV/AIDS treatment, and many argue that efforts to reduce new infections should become the central focus of donor assistance. This report outlines basic facts related to global HIV/AIDS, including characteristics of the epidemic and U.S. legislation, programs, funding, and partnerships related to global HIV/AIDS. It concludes with a brief description of some of the major issues that might be considered by the 112th Congress as it responds to the disease.

INTRODUCTION

Over the past decade, the United States has recognized the human immunodeficiency virus and the acquired immune deficiency syndrome (HIV/AIDS) as a key foreign policy priority. Congressional authorization of the President's Emergency Plan for AIDS Relief (PEPFAR) in 2003 brought unprecedented attention and funding to the epidemic and established a new and central role for donor governments in the fight against HIV/AIDS, particularly regarding the provision of AIDS treatment. The United States remains the largest single donor for global HIV/AIDS efforts in the world, providing over 50% of all government donor funds. In recent years, despite the continued challenge of HIV/AIDS around the world, international funding for HIV/AIDS—including U.S. assistance—has begun to level off. This report provides information on key components of the HIV/AIDS epidemic and the U.S. response to HIV/AIDS.

DESCRIPTION OF HIV/AIDS

HIV is an infectious disease that damages human immune cells. The final stage of HIV is AIDS, which occurs when an individual's immune system is so damaged it can no longer fight off other infections. If left untreated, AIDS is fatal. HIV is spread through contact with the bloodstream or by passing through delicate mucous membranes, including the vagina, rectum, and urethra. Transmission primarily occurs in three ways: (1) unprotected sexual intercourse with an infected partner; (2) injections with a needle, syringe, or other equipment that has been used by an infected person; and (3) between a child and an infected mother, during pregnancy, birth, or breast-feeding. High-risk groups include sex workers, men who have sex with men, and injecting drug users.

GLOBAL HIV/AIDS STATISTICS[1]

Prevalence: Prevalence measures the number of people living with a disease. Since the beginning of the epidemic, almost 60 million people have been infected with HIV. As of 2009, there were 33.3 million people living with the virus. Women make up 52% of those living with HIV. The number of people living with HIV continues to rise as a combined result of new infections and improved access to antiretroviral treatment (ART) that have lowed AIDS-related mortality.

Incidence: Incidence measures the number of people who contract a disease within a given time period (usually one year). In 2009, 2.6 million people contracted HIV—7,100 new infections per day—including 370,000 children under the age of 15. New infections are thought to have peaked in 1996 at 3.5 million (Figure 1). Incidence has fallen by more than 25% in 33 countries between 2001 and 2009, including in 22 sub-Saharan African countries.

Mortality: HIV continues to be a leading cause of death worldwide and the number one killer in sub-Saharan Africa. By 2009, more than 26 million people had died of AIDS worldwide. In 2009, 1.8 million people died of AIDS, including roughly 260,000 children. AIDS-related deaths are thought to have peaked in 2004 at 2.2 million and declined since then due to the improved access to ART.

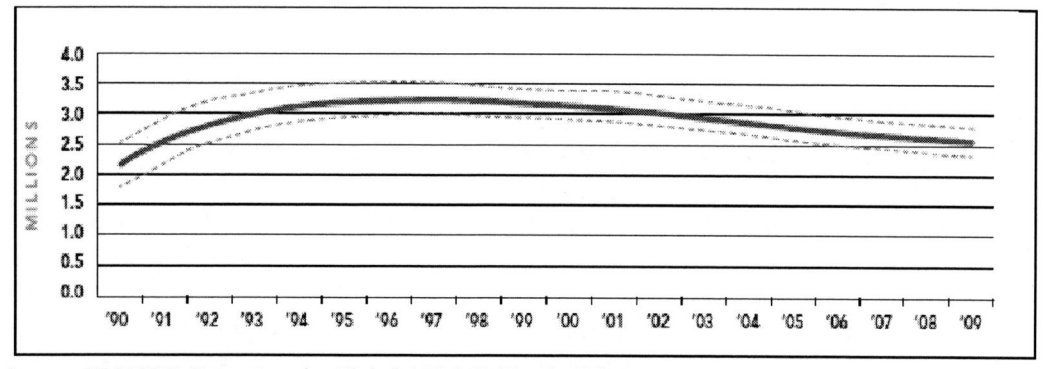

Source: UNAIDS, Report on the Global AIDS Epidemic, 2010, p. 16.
Notes: The dotted line represents high and low estimates of new infections each year.

Figure 1. Number of People Newly Infected with HIV, 1990-2009 (Millions per year).

REGIONAL DISTRIBUTION OF HIV/AIDS[2]

HIV/AIDS is a global phenomenon, but there are important regional and intra-regional differences in HIV prevalence, incidence, and mortality.

- Sub-Saharan Africa (SSA) is the region most affected by HIV/AIDS (**Figure 2**). As of 2009, an estimated 22.5 million people were living with HIV/AIDS in SSA, accounting for 68% of all people living with HIV worldwide. Nearly 90% of the estimated 16.9 million children who had lost one or both of their parents from AIDS-related deaths by the end of 2009 were in SSA. Southern Africa is home to the nine countries with the world's highest HIV prevalence rates worldwide and was home to an estimated 11.3 million people living with HIV in 2009. Swaziland has the world's highest prevalence rate (25.9%), and South Africa has the world's largest population with HIV (5.6 million). In 2009, about 1.8 million people in SSA contracted HIV and some 1.3 million people in the region died from AIDS.
- As of 2009, an estimated 4.9 million people were living with HIV in Asia, including 360,000 people who became infected in 2009. Also in 2009, approximately 300,000 AIDS-related deaths occurred in the region. Since 2000, the epidemic has remained somewhat stable in Asia, with HIV incidence peaking in the mid-1990s.
- As of 2009, an estimated 1.6 million people were living with HIV in Latin America and the Caribbean, including 109,000 people who became infected in 2009. In the region, the Bahamas has the highest prevalence rate, while Brazil has the largest population living with virus. Overall, the epidemic in Latin America has stabilized as has the rate of new infections in the Caribbean.
- Eastern Europe and Central Asia (EECA) has experienced the largest regional increase in HIV prevalence, most prominently in Russia and Ukraine. Since 2000, the number of people living with HIV in the region has almost tripled. As of 2009, an estimated 1.4 million people were living with HIV in EECA, including 130,000 people who were infected in 2009.

HIV/AIDS TREATMENT, CARE, AND PREVENTION

Treatment: Use of ART to treat HIV/AIDS has lowered the rate of AIDS-related deaths in much of the world. ART coverage—the percentage of people on ART among those in need—was 36% in 2009, up from 7% in 2003.[3] While lowering AIDS-related deaths, access to ART has also increased HIV prevalence around the world, as infected individuals are now living longer. ART also has some preventive benefits as it lowers viral loads, consequently reducing the likelihood of transmission.

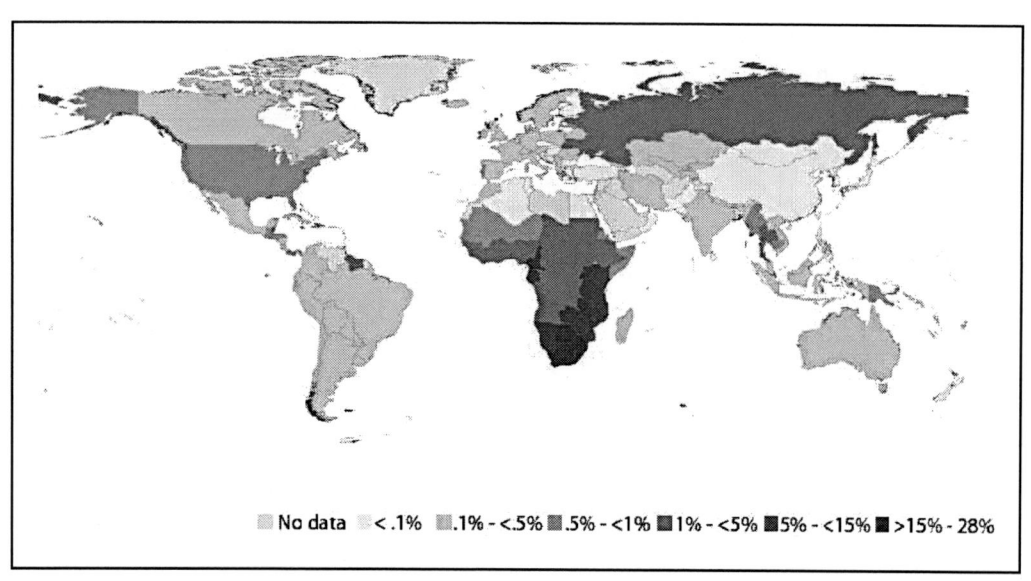

Source: UNAIDS, Report on the Global AIDS Epidemic, 2010, p. 23.
Notes: Prevalence rates measure the percentage of people living with HIV in each country.

Figure 2. Global Prevalence Rates of HIV, 2009.

Care Activities: Care for individuals infected and affected by HIV/AIDS constitutes a wide range of activities, including support for ART adherence, treatment of opportunistic infections, nutritional counseling, mental health services, prevention education, and livelihood activities, along with attention to orphans and vulnerable children.

Prevention Activities: A number of prevention efforts are being used to combat HIV/AIDS, including male circumcision, reduction of mother-to-child transmission (PMTCT), behavior change programs (including advocacy of abstinence, being faithful, and using condoms), HIV testing, blood supply safety programs, and harm reduction programs aimed at high-risk groups.

Prevention Research: Efforts to develop HIV preventive vaccines and microbicides— compounds that can be applied inside the vagina or rectum to protect against sexually transmitted infections—are underway. Results from a 2010 study in South Africa, funded in part by the United States, showed that the use of a microbicide was 39% effective in reducing a woman's risk of contracting HIV during sex.[4] Many health experts support microbicide research as it offers women vulnerable to violence and sexual coercion some degree of protection against HIV.

KEY U.S. LEGISLATION ON GLOBAL HIV/AIDS, 2003-2011

- On May 27, 2003, President George W. Bush signed into law the United States Leadership Against HIV/AIDS, Tuberculosis, and Malaria Act of 2003 (Leadership Act, P.L. 108-25). The Leadership Act authorized $15 billion for global HIV/AIDS,

TB, and malaria programs from FY2004 through FY2008. The act also authorized the creation of the Office of the Global AIDS Coordinator (OGAC) at the Department of State to oversee and coordinate all bilateral HIV/AIDS activities and funding.

As part of the act, Congress recommended the following distribution of HIV/AIDS funds:

- 15% of funds be used for palliative care, and
- 20% of funds be used for HIV/AIDS prevention efforts.

Congress further required the following distribution of HIV/AIDS funds for each fiscal year from FY2006 to FY2008:

- at least 55% of funds be used for AIDS treatment, of which at least 75% be used for the purchase and distribution of ART and at least 25% be used for related care;
- at least 33% of appropriated prevention funds be used for abstinence- until-marriage programs; and
- at least 10% of funds be spent on orphans and vulnerable children.

Finally, the act mandated that from FY2004 to FY2008, the United States contribution to the Global Fund to Fight AIDS, Tuberculosis, and Malaria (Global Fund, see, "Key Partners in the Response to Global HIV/AIDS") not exceed 33% of the total amount of funds contributed from all sources.

- On July 24, 2008, President Bush signed into law the Tom Lantos and Henry J. Hyde U.S. Global Leadership Against HIV/AIDS, Tuberculosis, and Malaria Reauthorization Act of 2008 (Lantos-Hyde Act, P.L. 110-293). The Lantos-Hyde Act authorized $48 billion for U.S. global HIV/AIDS, TB, and malaria efforts from FY2008 through FY2013, including $2 billion for the Global Fund in FY2008.

As part of the act, Congress removed the recommendations that 20% on funds be spent on prevention efforts and that 33% of these funds be used for abstinence-until-marriage programs, and required the following:

- for each fiscal year from FY2009 to FY2013, at least 10% of funds be spent on orphans and vulnerable children;
- for each fiscal year from FY2009 to FY2013, more than 50% of bilateral assistance be spent on treatment and care of individuals infected with HIV/AIDS;
- balanced funding for prevention activities including those that promote abstinence, delay of sexual debut, monogamy, fidelity, and partner reduction and country-specific implementation of such activities; and
- a report to Congress should less than 50% of prevention funds go to activities promoting abstinence, delay of sexual debut, monogamy, fidelity, and partner reduction in any country with a generalized epidemic.

U.S. GLOBAL HIV/AIDS PROGRAMS

In 1999, the 106th Congress authorized resources to support a proposal by the Clinton Administration to broaden U.S. activities related to global HIV/AIDS through the Leadership and Investment in Fighting an Epidemic (LIFE) initiative. LIFE sought to address HIV/AIDS in 14 African countries and in India and represented the first time agencies other than the United States Agency for International Development (USAID) were included in the U.S. response to HIV/AIDS. President George W. Bush launched two initiatives that built on the LIFE initiative. In 2002, President Bush announced the International Mother and Child HIV Prevention Initiative, which focused on preventing mother-to-child transmission of HIV in 12 African countries and in two Caribbean countries. In 2003, President Bush announced PEPFAR, proposing that the United States spend $15 billion over the course of five years to combat HIV/AIDS. Both the LIFE initiative and the International Mother and Child HIV Prevention Initiative were replaced by PEPFAR.

PEPFAR significantly increased attention to and funding for global HIV/AIDS. The President proposed that the majority of the funds ($9 billion) be concentrated in 15 focus countries, including 12 in sub-Saharan Africa. The proposal also allocated $5 billion to research and to other bilateral HIV/AIDS programs and $1 billion for contributions in FY2004 to the Global Fund.

PEPFAR represents the largest commitment by any country toward an international health issue. At the time it was established, health experts were debating whether the international community had a responsibility to provide ART to HIV-positive people in developing countries and whether they could be safely administered in such environments. PEPFAR responded to calls from those advocating treatment for the world's poor and demonstrated that ART could be effectively provided in low-resource settings.

Through the Leadership Act, Congress authorized the establishment of the Office of the Global AIDS Coordinator (OGAC), at the Department of State. OGAC oversees and coordinates all U.S. spending on bilateral global HIV/AIDS activities implemented by various agencies (see "PEPFAR Implementing Agencies"), as well as contributions to multilateral organizations.

President Barack Obama has committed to continued support for PEPFAR, while working to transition PEPFAR from an emergency plan to a long-term and sustainable approach to global HIV/AIDS. On May 5, 2009, the President announced the six-year, $63 billion Global Health Initiative (GHI), a new effort to develop a comprehensive U.S. global health strategy. The GHI calls for a more integrated U.S. response to global health issues and for a shift in U.S. global health strategy from one focused on specific diseases to a more comprehensive approach to health. PEPFAR is the central component of the GHI and accounts for over 60% of the President's FY2012 budget proposal. As part of the GHI, PEPFAR has committed to supporting the following goals from FY2010 through FY2014:

- prevention of more than 12 million new HIV infections;
- treatment of more than 4 million people living with HIV/AIDS;
- care for more than 12 million people, including 5 million orphans and vulnerable children; and
- training and retention of more than 140,000 new heath care workers.[5]

PEPFAR IMPLEMENTING AGENCIES

PEPFAR programs are led by OGAC at the State Department and implemented by various U.S. agencies and departments, including the following:

- **U.S. Agency for International Development:** USAID supports HIV/AIDS programs in nearly 100 countries. These programs focus on providing treatment, care, and support to people infected with HIV/AIDS; strengthening primary health care systems; providing training, technical assistance, and commodities that reduce HIV transmission; reducing high-risk behaviors; and supporting international partnerships.
- **Centers for Diseases Control and Prevention (CDC):** CDC's Global AIDS Program (GAP) operates in 38 countries and three regional programs. CDC HIV/AIDS programs assist ministries of health and local implementing organizations to implement HIV/AIDS prevention programs, analyze program impact and cost effectiveness, and build the capacity of public workforce, as well as public health information, laboratory, and management systems.
- **National Institutes of Health (NIH):** NIH supports HIV/AIDS research and training in 90 countries. This research focuses on tools to prevent HIV transmission, such as vaccines and microbicides; strategies to prevent mother-to-child transmission; and approaches to treating HIV and its associated opportunistic infections and co-infections in resource poor settings.
- **Health Resources and Services Administration (HRSA):** HRSA's HIV/AIDS strategy focuses on health system strengthening and improvements in human resources for health. HRSA runs HIV/AIDS programs in more than 25 countries that support rapid roll-out of ART, education and training for health workers, and innovative approaches to health data collection and evaluation.
- **U.S. Food and Drug Administration (FDA):** FDA ensures the availability of safe and effective AIDS treatment. Since 2004, FDA has supported an accelerated review process for ARTs, including generic drugs and fixed dose combination drugs (FDCs)—multiple antiretroviral drugs combined into a single pill—for PEPFAR programs. As of 2008, 80 generic ART formulations, including 16 FDCs, had been approved or tentatively approved by FDA.
- **Department of Defense (DOD):** DOD operates HIV/AIDS programs in 73 countries. DOD's primary role under PEPFAR is to support military-to-military HIV/AIDS prevention, treatment, and care efforts; assist in the development of military-specific HIV/AIDS policies; and provide HIV/AIDS counseling, testing, and care for military families. DOD also provides HIV prevention scientific and technical assistance to non-military PEPFAR programs. The DOD HIV/AIDS Prevention Program (DHAPP) manages DOD's HIV/AIDS programs for foreign militaries and oversees the use of PEPFAR funds by other DOD organizations.
- **Department of Labor (DOL):** DOL implements HIV/AIDS programs in over 23 countries that facilitate the development of comprehensive workplace-based HIV prevention and education programs; assist governments, employers, and trade unions to develop and disseminate workplace policy countering stigma and discrimination;

and support collaboration between government, business, and labor in countering HIV/AIDS.

- **Peace Corps:** Peace Corps volunteers support community-based HIV/AIDS care and prevention efforts in 77 countries. In FY2009, 21% of Peace Corps volunteer projects were related to HIV/AIDS and 25 Peace Corps posts received direct PEPFAR funding, while other posts benefited from activities organized by the headquarters using central PEPFAR funding.
- **U.S. Department of Commerce (DOC):** DOC creates and disseminates sector-specific strategies to inform HIV trade advisory committees on how the private sector can help combat HIV/AIDS. The U.S. Census Bureau also contributes to PEPFAR by assisting with data management and analysis, estimating infections averted, and supporting mapping of country-level activities.

U.S. GLOBAL HIV/AIDS ASSISTANCE FUNDS

Congress provides funds for HIV/AIDS assistance to several U.S. agencies through a number of appropriations vehicles: State-Foreign Operations (State-Foreign Ops); Labor, Health and Human Services and Education (Labor-HHS); and Department of Defense (Defense) (**Figure 3**). **Table 1** details all U.S. funding for global HIV/AIDS since FY2004.

- **State-Foreign Operations Appropriations:** The majority of PEPFAR funds are appropriated through State-Foreign Operations to the Department of State. In FY2010, Congress appropriated approximately 81% of all global HIV/AIDS funds to the Department of State. As the coordinator of global HIV/AIDS activities, the Department of State transfers the bulk of these funds to implementing agencies in support of bilateral HIV/AIDS programs. Per congressional proviso, the Department also uses some of these funds to make contributions to other organizations that combat global HIV/AIDS, including the Global Fund. Congress also appropriates funds to USAID for bilateral HIV/AIDS activities through State-Foreign Operations appropriations.
- **Labor, Health and Human Services, and Education Appropriations:** Congress appropriates funds for global HIV/AIDS activities to HHS agencies, including CDC and NIH, through Labor-HHS appropriations. Congress provides a second portion of the U.S. contribution to the Global Fund through Labor-HHS. Congress used to appropriate funds to DOL for bilateral HIV/AIDS activities, but it has not done so since FY2005. DOL's HIV/AIDS programs are now supported through transfers from the Department of State.
- **Department of Defense Appropriations:** Congress also appropriates funds to DOD for bilateral HIV/AIDS programs through DOD appropriations.

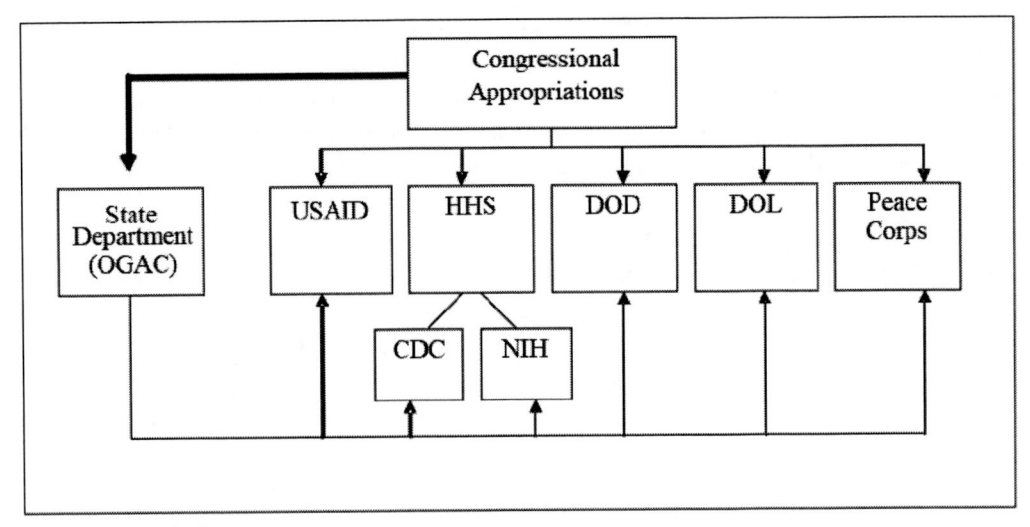

Source: CRS analysis.

Figure 3. PEPFAR Organizational Chart: Appropriations.

Table 1. U.S. Bilateral Funding for Global HIV/AIDS: FY2004-FY2012 ($ Millions, Current)

Program/ Agency	FY2004 Actual	FY2005 Actual	FY2006 Actual	FY2007 Actual	FY2008 Actual	FY2009 Actual	FY2010 Estimate	FY2004-FY2010 TOTAL	FY2011 Request	FY2012 Request
USAID	555.5	384.7	373.8	345.9	371.1	350.0	350.0	2,731.0	350.0	350.0
State	488.1	1,373.9	1,777.1	2,869.0	4,116.4	4,559.0	4,609.0	19,792.5	4,800.0	4,641.9
Of which, UNAIDS	*0.0*	*27.0*	*29.7*	*30.0*	*35.0*	*40.0*	*43.0*	*204.7*	*45.0*	*45.0*
FMF[a]	1.5	2.0	2.0	1.6	1.0	n/s	n/s	n/s	n/s	n/s
CDC	266.9	123.8	122.6	121	118.9	118.9	119.0	991.1	118.1	118.0
NIH	317.2	369.5	373.0	361.7	411.7	451.7	485.6	2,770.4	470.6	489.4
DOL	9.9	2.0	0.0	0.0	0.0	0.0	0.0	11.8	0.0	0.0
DOD	4.3	7.5	5.2	0.0	8.0	8.0	10.0	43.0	0.0	n/s
TOTAL Bilateral HIV/AIDS	**1,643.4**	**2,263.4**	**2,653.7**	**3,699.2**	**5,027.1**	**5,487.6**	**5,573.6**	**26,348.0**	**5,738.7**	**5,599.3**

Source: Compiled by CRS from Congressional Budget Justifications and appropriations legislation.

Note: FY2011 Funding is currently provided under a continuing resolution at FY2010-enacted levels until March 4, 2011. "n/s" stands for "not specified" and "n/a" stands for "not available."

a. Foreign Military Financing (FMF) funds are used to purchase equipment for DOD HIV/AIDS Programs.

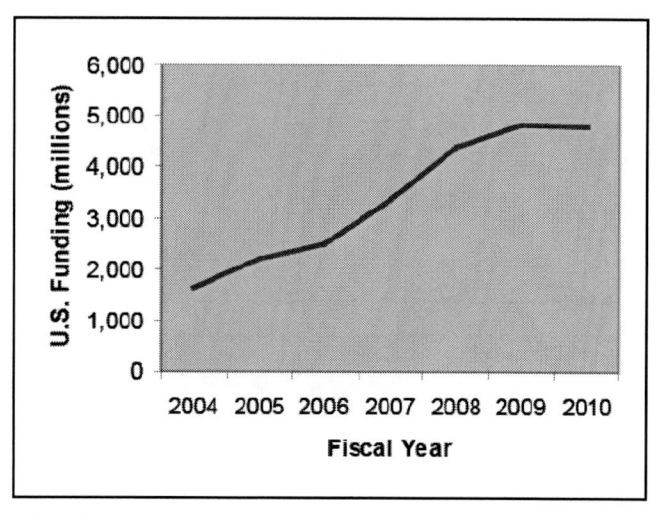

Source: Compiled by CRS from Congress Budget Justifications.

Figure 4. U.S. Funding for Bilateral Global HIV/AIDS Programs in Constant Dollars: FY2004-FY2010 ($ millions, constant).

Since the establishment of PEPFAR, U.S. funding for global HIV/AIDS has increased each year, with the largest increases between FY2004 and FY2008. U.S. funding for bilateral global HIV/AIDS programs has been largely level since FY2008 (Figure 4).

The United States also supports global HIV/AIDS programs through contributions to the Global Fund, an international financing mechanism for the response to HIV/AIDS, TB, and malaria (**Table 2**). U.S. contributions to the Global Fund support grants for HIV/AIDS, TB, and malaria. The Global Fund has historically directed approximately 61% of its funds for HIV/AIDS efforts. [6] The United States is the single largest donor to the Global Fund.

Table 2. U.S. Appropriations for the Global Fund: FY2004-FY2012 ($ millions, current)

Program/ Agency	FY2004 Actual	FY2005 Actual	FY2006 Actual	FY2007 Actual	FY2008 Actual	FY2009 Actual	FY2010 Estimate	FY2004-FY2010 TOTAL	FY2011 Request	FY2012 Request
USAID Global Fund	397.6	248.0	247.5	247.5	0.0	100.0	0.0	1,240.6	0.0	0.0
FY2004 Carryover	-87.8	87.8	n/a	n/a	n/a	n/a	n/a	n/a	n/a	n/a
State Global Fund	0.0	0.0	198.0	377.5	545.5	600.0	750.0	2,471.0	700.0	1,000.0
HHS Global Fund	149.1	99.2	99.0	99.0	294.8	300.0	300.0	1,341.1	300.0	300.0
TOTAL Global Fund	**458.9**	**435.0**	**544.5**	**724.0**	**840.3**	**1,000.0**	**1,050.0**	**5,052.7**	**1,000.0**	**1,300.0**

Source: Compiled by CRS from appropriations legislation.

Notes: In the "FY2004 Carryover" row, "n/a" is used to reflect requirements in the U.S. Leadership Act, which stipulates that U.S. contributions to the Fund not exceed 33% of Fund contributions from all sources. FY2005 Consolidated Appropriations (P.L. 108-447) added this amount to the 2005 contribution, subject to the same 33% limitation.

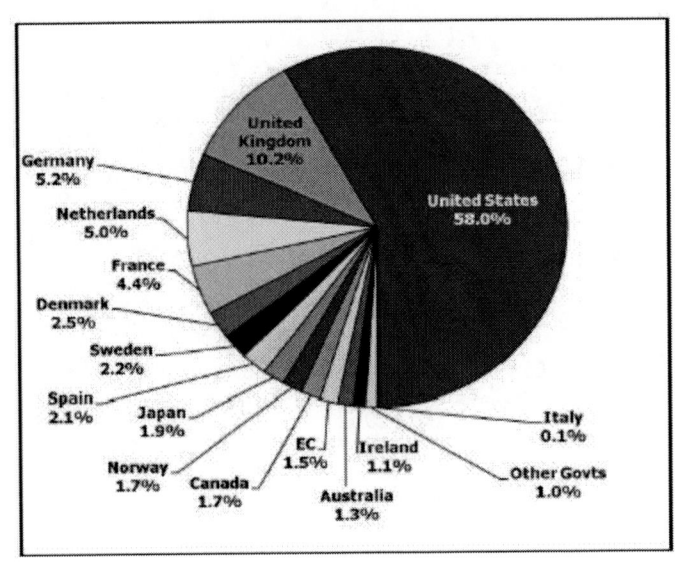

Source: UNAIDS and Kaiser Family Foundation, Financing the Response to AIDS in Low- and Middle-Income Countries: International Assistance from the G8, European Commission and Other Donor Governments in 2009, July 2010, p. 5.
Notes: EC stands for European Commission.

Figure 5. Donor Government HIV/AIDS Assistance, as Share of Total Disbursements, 2009 (Percent of $ billions, current).

In low-income countries, 88% of total spending on HIV/AIDS is from international sources, just over three-quarters of which is from bilateral donors, with the remaining quarter from multilateral donors. In 2009, U.S. funds made up over half of all donor government disbursements for global HIV/AIDS (**Figure 5**) and 27% of global HIV/AIDS funds from all sources, including donor and domestic governments, multilateral organizations, and the private sector.[7] When standardized to correspond to gross domestic product (GDP) per $1 million spent, six European countries spend more than the United States on global HIV/AIDS.[8]

KEY PARTNERS IN THE RESPONSE TO GLOBAL HIV/AIDS

The United States works with a range of partners to combat HIV/AIDS, including other national governments, multilateral organizations, non-governmental organizations (NGOs), and the private sector. Through authorizing legislation and annual appropriations, Congress provides funds to several multilateral organizations and international research initiatives who contribute to the fight against HIV/AIDS, including the Global Fund and the United Nations Joint Program on HIV/AIDS (UNAIDS).

- **The Global Fund:** The Global Fund was established in 2002 as a public-private partnership to provide financial support for global responses to HIV/AIDS, TB, and malaria. The United States contributes more to the Global Fund than any other country. By the end of 2009, the Global Fund had committed to grant roughly \$10.8 billion for HIV/AIDS programs in 140 countries.[9]

- **UNAIDS:** UNAIDS is the main advocate for United Nations (U.N.) action on HIV/AIDS and is responsible for coordinating HIV/AIDS activities implemented by nine agencies, including U.N. Children's Fund (UNICEF); U.N. Development Program (UNDP); International Labor Organization (ILO); U.N. Population Fund (UNFPA); U.N. Office on Drugs and Crime (UNODC); U.N. Educational, Scientific and Cultural Organization (UNESCO); World Food Program (WFP); World Health Organization (WHO); and the World Bank. The United States is one of the largest contributors to UNAIDS. UNAIDS oversees a wide range of HIV/AIDS activities, which include efforts to reduce transmission of HIV; ensure access to ART; prevent death from HIV/TB co-infection; empower men who have sex with men; remove punitive law, policies, and practices that block effective responses to AIDS; reduce sexual and gender-based violence; and empower young people to protect themselves from HIV.

KEY ISSUES IN GLOBAL HIV/AIDS

The 112th Congress will likely be faced with a number of issues regarding the U.S. response to global HIV/AIDS, including how much assistance to provide and how to best apportion global HIV/AIDS funds. Given the United States' central role in the fight against HIV/AIDS, many experts assert that the future direction of the U.S. response to HIV/AIDS will have significant implications for the global response to HIV/AIDS as a whole. The 112th Congress may consider the following issues as it considers the U.S. response to global HIV/AIDS:

- **Treatment efforts:** Without a vaccine or cure to HIV, people continue to contract HIV and require lifelong treatment. As such, despite efforts by the international community to expand access to treatment, the number of people in need of ART outpaces treatment resources. Global health experts have increasingly debated the sustainability of offering HIV/AIDS treatment and whether treatment should continue to be the central focus of donor assistance.
- **Prevention efforts:** There is widespread support within the global health community for intensifying prevention efforts, particularly in light of the persistent need for HIV/AIDS treatments. At the same time, experts disagree on what prevention efforts are most effective, how to measure the success of any one prevention activity, and how to incentivize leaders of developing countries to increase financial investment in prevention, particularly given its less immediate and dramatic results when compared with treatment.
- **Health System Strengthening:** Many global health experts argue that an effective long-term approach to global HIV/AIDS requires efforts to strengthen health systems (HSS) in low- and middle-income countries. However, there is little consensus within the global health community over how to define, implement, and measure

HSS activities, and over whether PEPFAR has had a beneficial or detrimental impact on the broader functioning of health systems.

- **Country ownership:** Donor governments have increasingly supported the concept of country ownership as a way to promote sustainable and country-appropriate responses to the epidemic. To this end, PEPFAR programs have begun to implement "Partnership Frameworks" with partner countries to clarify joint goals and strategies. A number of issues related to country ownership are being debated within donor governments, including how to best align donor priorities and country priorities and how to maintain effective levels of oversight while shifting control to host governments.

End Notes

[1] All data in this section is from Joint United Nations Program on HIV/AIDS (UNAIDS), *Report on the Global AIDS Epidemic*, 2010, http://www.unaids.org/documents/20101123_GlobalReport_em.pdf.

[2] All data in this section is from UNAIDS, *Report on the Global AIDS Epidemic*, 2010.

[3] UNAIDS, *Report on the Global AIDS Epidemic*, 2010.

[4] Center for the AIDS Program of Research in South Africa (CAPRISA), *Study of Microbicide Gel Shows Reduced Risk of HIV and Herpes Infection in Women*, July 20, 2010, http://www.caprisa.org/joomla/index.php/component/ content/article/1/226.

[5] The President's Emergency Plan For AIDS Relief, *The U.S. President's Emergency Plan for AIDS Relief: Five-Year Strategy*, Office of the Global AIDS Coordinator, Department of State, 2009, http://www.pepfar.gov/strategy/.

[6] The Global Fund to Fight AIDS, Tuberculosis and Malaria, *Distribution of Funding After 7 Rounds*, http://www.theglobalfund.org/en/distributionfunding/?lang=en#disease.

[7] UNAIDS, *Report on the Global AIDS Epidemic*, 2010.

[8] UNAIDS and Kaiser Family Foundation, Financing the Response to AIDS in Low- and Middle-Income Countries: International Assistance from the G8, European Commission and Other Donor Governments in 2009, July 2010, http://www.kff.org/hivaids/upload/7347-06.pdf.

[9] The Global Fund to Fight AIDS, Tuberculosis, and Malaria, *Innovation and Impact: Results Summary*, 2010, http://www.theglobalfund.org/documents/replenishment/2010/Progress_Report_Summary_2010_en.pdf.

In: Global HIV/AIDS Threat and the U.S. Response
Editor: David R. Carmody

ISBN: 978-1-61324-568-2
© 2011 Nova Science Publishers, Inc.

Chapter 2

THE U.S. PRESIDENT'S EMERGENCY PLAN FOR AIDS RELIEF (FIVE-YEAR STRATEGY)

David R. Carmody

I. EXECUTIVE SUMMARY OF PEPFAR'S STRATEGY

Launched in 2003 by President George W. Bush, PEPFAR holds a place in history as the largest effort by any nation to combat a single disease. In the first five years of the program, PEPFAR focused on establishing and scaling up prevention, care and treatment programs. It achieved success in expanding access to HIV prevention, care and treatment in low-resource settings. During its first phase, PEPFAR supported the provision of treatment to more than 2 million people, care to more than 10 million people, including more than 4 million orphans and vulnerable children, and prevention of mother-to-child treatment services during nearly 16 million pregnancies.

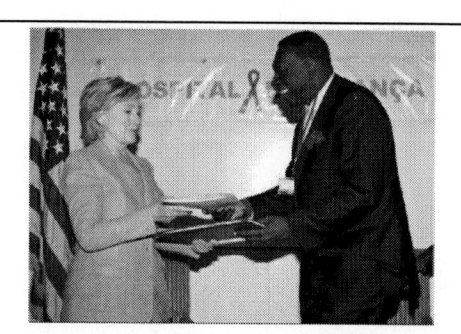

On August 10, 2009, Secretary of State Hillary Rodham Clinton and Angolan Minister of External Relations Assunção Afonso dos Anjos signed the "Partnership Framework between the Government of the Republic of Angola and the Government of the United States of America to Combat HIV/AIDS for 2009 – 2013." The Partnership Framework provides a five-year joint strategic plan for cooperation between the Government of Angola and the U.S. Government, with participation of other stakeholders, to support achievement of the goals of Angola's HIV National Strategic Plan for 2007-2010.

New Directions

This global epidemic requires a comprehensive, multisectoral approach that expands access to prevention, care and treatment. As PEPFAR works to build upon its successes, it will focus on transitioning from an emergency response to promoting sustainable country programs.

Sustainable programs must be country-owned and country-driven. Given that the AIDS epidemic represents a shared global burden among nations, the next phase of PEPFAR represents an opportunity for the United States to support shared responsibility with partner countries. To seize this opportunity, PEPFAR is supporting countries in taking leadership of the responses to their epidemics. In addition, to support an expanded collective impact at the country level, PEPFAR is increasing collaboration with multilateral organizations.

Sustainable programs must address HIV/AIDS within a broader health and development context. PEPFAR must be responsive to the overall health needs faced by people living with HIV/AIDS (PLWHA), their families, and their communities, linking the HIV response to a diverse array of global health challenges. As a component of the Global Health Initiative, PEPFAR will be carefully and purposefully integrated with other health and development programs. Integration expands country capacity to address a broader array of health demands and to respond to new and emerging challenges presented by HIV. Strategic coordination furthers the reach of bilateral assistance, leverages the work of multilateral organizations, promotes country ownership, and increases the sustainability of national health programs.

Sustainable programs must build upon our strengths and increase efficiencies. PEPFAR is renewing its emphasis on a "whole of government" response, ensuring that agencies focus on core competencies and better coordination to maximize the effectiveness of U.S. Government (USG) assistance. It is also identifying and implementing efficiencies in its work at both field and headquarters levels to ensure value for money. To build upon the strengths of proven programs, PEPFAR is scaling up effective interventions, particularly in prevention. Finally, it is working to ensure that increased access to coverage is accompanied by an emphasis on quality of services.

PEPFAR's Goals

1. Transition from an emergency response to promotion of sustainable country programs.
2. Strengthen partner government capacity to lead the response to this epidemic and other health demands.
3. Expand prevention, care, and treatment in both concentrated and generalized epidemics.
4. Integrate and coordinate HIV/AIDS programs with broader global health and development programs to maximize impact on health systems.
5. Invest in innovation and operations research to evaluate impact, improve service delivery and maximize outcomes.

PEPFAR's Targets from Fiscal Year (FY) 2010- FY 2014:[*]

Prevention

- support the prevention of more than 12 million new HIV infections;
- ensure that every partner country with a generalized epidemic has both 80% coverage of testing for pregnant women at the national level, and 85% coverage of antiretroviral drug (ARV) prophylaxis and treatment, as indicated, of women found to be HIV-infected;
- double the number of at-risk babies born HIV-free, from the 240,000 babies of HIV-positive mothers who were born HIV-negative during the first five years of PEPFAR;
- in every partner country with a generalized epidemic, provide 100% of youth in PEPFAR prevention programs with comprehensive and correct knowledge of the ways HIV/AIDS is transmitted and ways to protect themselves, consistent with Millennium Development Goal indicators in this area.

Care and Support and Treatment

- provide direct support for more than 4 million people on treatment, more than doubling the number of people directly supported on treatment during the first five years of PEPFAR;[*]
- support care for more than 12 million people, including 5 million orphans and vulnerable children (OVCs); and
- ensure that every partner country with a generalized epidemic reaches a threshold of 65% coverage for early infant diagnosis at the national level, and testing of 80% of older children of HIV-positive mothers, with increased referrals and linkages to care and treatment.

Sustainability

- support training and retention of more than 140,000 new health care workers to strengthen health systems;
- in order to support country ownership, ensure that in each country with a major PEPFAR investment (greater than $5 million), the partner government leads efforts to evaluate and define needs and roles in the national response; and
- ensure that in every partner country with a Partnership Framework, each country will change policies to address the larger structural conditions, such as gender-based violence, stigma, or low male partner involvement, which contribute to the spread of the epidemic.

Programmatic Strategy

In this second phase of PEPFAR, a new program strategy is underway that supports the Administration's overall emphasis on improving health outcomes, increasing program sustainability and integration, and strengthening health systems. Some of these changes are

---

[*] For more information on PEPFAR's data collection, please visit: *www.pepfar.gov/2009results/*.

already being implemented with planning and programming for FY 2010. Over the next year, PEPFAR will be working closely with country teams in order to translate, prioritize, and implement this strategy in a manner appropriate to the country context. More information on the broader strategic framework for PEPFAR activities can be found in the strategy annexes which will be made available at *www.pepfar.gov/strategy*.

Prevention

Prevention remains the paramount challenge of the HIV epidemic, and the major priority for the next five years of PEPFAR. Successful prevention programs require a combination of evidence-based, mutually reinforcing biomedical, behavioral, and structural interventions. PEPFAR is expanding its prevention activities with an emphasis on the following:

- Working with countries to track and reassess the epidemiology of the epidemic, in order to fashion a prevention response based on best available and most recent data;
- Emphasizing prevention strategies that have been proven effective and targeting interventions to most at-risk populations with high incidence rates; and
- Increasing emphasis on supporting and evaluating innovative and promising prevention methods.

Linking HIV/AIDS to Women's and Children's Health

According to the World Health Organization (WHO), AIDS is the leading cause of death among women aged 15-44 worldwide.[1] Nearly 60% of those living with HIV in sub-Saharan Africa are women.[2] UNICEF estimates that nearly 12 million children in sub-Saharan Africa have lost one or both parents to HIV/AIDS.[3] Women and children living with HIV also face other conditions, ranging from inadequate access to family planning to lack of antenatal care to the need for food and nutrition support. As part of its overall prevention, care and support, and treatment efforts, PEPFAR is leveraging and linking HIV services to broader delivery mechanisms that improve health outcomes for women and children. Some of these activities include:

- Increasing investment in prevention of mother-tochild transmission to meet 80% coverage levels in HIV testing and counseling of pregnant women and 85% coverage levels of ARV prophylaxis for those women who test positive;
- Increasing the proportion of HIV-infected infants and children who receive treatment commensurate to their representation in a country's overall epidemic, helping countries to meet national coverage levels of 65% for early infant diagnosis, and doubling the number of at-risk babies born HIV-free;
- Expanding integration of HIV prevention, care and support, and treatment services with family planning and reproductive health services, so that women living with HIV can access necessary care, and so that all women know how to protect themselves from HIV infection;
- Strengthening the ability of families and communities to provide supportive services, such as food, nutrition, education, livelihood and vocational training, to orphans and vulnerable children; and

- Expanding PEPFAR's commitment to cross-cutting integration of gender equity in its programs and policies, with a new focus on addressing and reducing gender-based violence.

Treatment

PEPFAR's treatment programs provide essential medications to more than two million people. PEPFAR also contributes to the strengthening of the health systems needed to deliver these drugs in low-resource settings. In addition, PEPFAR serves populations with special treatment needs, like children. Together, all global efforts support approximately four million people on antiretroviral treatment, but at least five million more are still in need of ARV drugs.[4] This figure will likely double with the recent revision of WHO recommendations for treatment initiation. As part of its reauthorization, PEPFAR was charged with supporting increased treatment commensurate with increased appropriations and efficiencies realized. PEPFAR's treatment strategy over the next five years emphasizes the following activities:

- Directly supporting more than 4 million people on treatment, more than doubling the number of patients directly supported by PEPFAR in its first five years;
- Scaling up treatment with a particular focus on serving the sickest individuals, pregnant women and those with HIV/TB coinfection;
- Increasing support for country-level treatment capacity by strengthening health systems and expanding the number of trained health workers; and
- Working with countries and international organizations to develop a shared global response to the burden of treatment costs in the developing world, and assisting countries in achieving their defined treatment targets.

Health Systems Strengthening

PEPFAR has had a positive impact on the capacity of country health systems to address the WHO's six building blocks of health systems functions. However, the program to date has not placed a deliberate focus on the strategic strengthening of health systems. In its next phase, PEPFAR is working to enhance the ability of governments to manage their epidemics, respond to broader health needs impacting affected communities, and address new and emerging health concerns. PEPFAR now emphasizes the incorporation of health systems strengthening goals into its prevention, care and treatment portfolios. Doing so will help to reduce the burden of HIV/AIDS on the overall health system. Planned activities include the following:

- Training and retention of health care workers, managers, administrators, health economists, and other civil service employees critical to all functions of a health system;
- Implementing a new health systems framework to assist country teams in targeting and leveragingPEPFAR activities in support of a stronger country
- Supporting efforts to identify and implement harmonized health systems measurement tools; and
- Coordinating USG activities across multilateral partners to leverage and enhance broader health system strengthening activities.

Country Ownership

PEPFAR's commitment to the principles of country ownership highlights a new focus on engaging in true partnership with countries. These partnerships pave the way for new approaches to foreign assistance based upon principles and directions common to partner country plans and USG objectives. Over the next five years, PEPFAR's emphasis on country ownership will include:

- Continuing bilateral engagement through its Partnership Frameworks and other efforts to promote and develop a more sustainable response to the local epidemic, whether concentrated or generalized;
- Ensuring that the services PEPFAR supports are aligned with the national plans of partner governments and integrated with existing health care delivery systems;
- Strengthening engagement with diplomatic efforts at all levels of government to raise the profile and dialogue around the AIDS epidemic and its linkages with broader health and development issues;
- Expanding technical assistance and mentoring to country governments, in order to support a capable cadre of professionals to carry out the tasks necessary for a functioning health system; and
- Partnering with governments through bilateral, regional and multilateral mechanisms to support and facilitate South-to-South technical assistance.

Integration

As the largest component of President Obama's Global Health Initiative, PEPFAR is actively working to enhance the integration of quality interventions with the broader health and development programs of the USG, country partners, multilateral organizations, and other donors.

Through activities like co-location of services and expanded training of health care workers, PEPFAR can expand access to overall care and support for infected and affected individuals. As noted earlier, a particular focus of PEPFAR's integration is to expand access to care for women and children. PEPFAR is also emphasizing engagement with broader health and development programs. Some examples include:

- Expanding HIV/TB integration by ensuring that PLWHA are routinely screened and treated for TB, and that people with TB are tested for HIV and referred, with follow up, for appropriate prophylaxis and treatment;
- Linking PEPFAR food and nutrition programs with the new USG Global Hunger and Food Security Initiative;
- Expanding partnerships with education, economic strengthening, microfinance, and vocational training programs; and
- Promoting accountable and responsive governance through increased bilateral engagement and capacity building with partner governments.

Multilateral Engagement

PEPFAR is part of a shared global responsibility to address global health needs. Its success has been closely linked to the success of newer multilateral initiatives such as the

Global Fund for AIDS, Tuberculosis and Malaria (Global Fund), and long-standing multilateral organizations including the Joint United Nations Programme on HIV/AIDS (UNAIDS) and WHO. PEPFAR is expanding its multilateral engagement with the goal of strengthening these institutions and leveraging their work to maximize the impact of PEPFAR. PEPFAR's multilateral engagement includes a new emphasis on the following:

- Supporting the Global Fund's efforts to improve oversight, grant performance, and its overall grant architecture in order to position it as a key partner for PEPFAR;
- Supporting UNAIDS efforts to mobilize global action and facilitate adoption of country-level changes that allow for rapid scale-up of key interventions;
- Negotiating a strategic framework for greater PEPFAR-WHO engagement; and
- Increasing coordination with multilateral development banks to improve the performance of health systems investments and better integrate with their broader economic development efforts.

Monitoring, Metrics and Research

PEPFAR's work can and should be systematically studied and analyzed to help inform public health and clinical practice. PEPFAR is not a research organization, but is expanding its current partnerships with implementers, researchers, and academic organizations to improve the science that guides this work. As PEPFAR transitions to support sustainable, country-led systems, it will improve efforts to contribute to the evidence base around HIV interventions, as well as broader health systems strengthening and integration. Over its next phase, PEPFAR will support the following new initiatives:

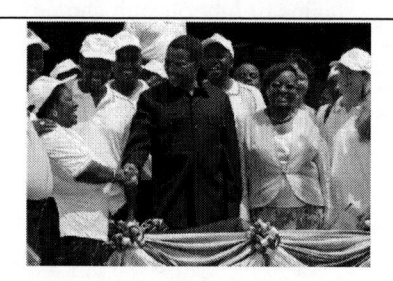

Tanzanian President Jakaya Kikwete launched the PEPFAR-supported Angaza Zaidi HIV counseling and testing program in April 2009. This program provides urban and rural communities in Tanzania with HIV counseling and testing services, post-test support groups, and referrals for HIV- positive individuals to care and treatment facilities.

- Building the country capacity necessary to implement and maintain a fully comprehensive data use strategy;
- Reducing the reporting burden on partner countries and supporting transition to a single, streamlined national monitoring and evaluation system; and
- Working to expand publicly available data.

II. PEPFAR's FIVE-YEAR STRATEGY

Introduction

The HIV/AIDS epidemic that confronted the world at the beginning of this decade was a humanitarian crisis of a magnitude never before faced in modern history. Despite significant advances in treatment and care in countries like the United States, the life-saving medications available in developed countries were largely inaccessible in developing nations. In 2001, fewer than 50,000 people living with HIV in sub-Saharan Africa had access to antiretroviral medication. As a result, many national health systems were overwhelmed. HIV-related needs absorbed almost all health care services available. Hospitals were packed with people dying from AIDS, spilling forth from beds onto floors and into hallways. Demoralized health care workers turned away severely ill patients, sending them home to die, because they had no treatment to offer.

The impact of the epidemic extended far beyond the health sector and those who were sick. AIDS created millions of orphans and robbed children of the stability and love of their parents. Many youth were forced to drop out of school and assume caregiver status for ailing parents and younger siblings. In addition, the AIDS epidemic paralyzed economies. At the country level, AIDS decimated national gains in economic growth. At a community level, AIDS created poverty among widows and families, and devastated schools, factories, armies and businesses whose employees were dying more quickly than they could be replaced. Adults were dying from AIDS during the time in their life when they should have been at the peak of their earning and production potential. Life expectancy in sub-Saharan Africa overall plummeted, reversing hard-earned gains of other health and development programs.

In 2003, President George W. Bush and a bipartisan Congress created the U.S. President's Emergency Plan for AIDS Relief to address this growing crisis. This program holds a place in the history of public health as the largest commitment by any nation to combat a single disease, establishing and expanding the infrastructure necessary to deliver prevention, care, and treatment services in low- resource settings. PEPFAR works to address HIV/AIDS in countries with a diversity of need in these service areas. It operates both in countries where epidemics are concentrated among specific populations and those where HIV infection occurs among the general population. In many countries where HIV infection prevalence rates are above 1% - the accepted threshold for generalized epidemics – PEPFAR also works to address the epidemic among most at-risk populations.

The achievements of PEPFAR are remarkable by any measure. From its creation through September 30, 2008, PEPFAR received total funding of more than $18 billion. In FY 2009, the USG invested more than $6.4 billion in bilateral HIV/AIDS programming and the Global Fund to Fight AIDS, Tuberculosis, and Malaria. In FY 2009 alone, PEPFAR directly supported more than 2.4 million patients on treatment, and more than 11 million people with care and support programs.[*] During its first five years, PEPFAR's efforts around prevention of motherto-child transmission programs allowed nearly 240,000 babies of HIV-positive mothers to be born HIV-free. In addition, during this time, more than 4 million orphans and vulnerable children were assisted by the program. PEPFAR also supported over 16,000

---

[*] For more information on PEPFAR's data collection, please visit: www.pepfar.gov/2009results/.

laboratories, approximately 3.7 million training and retraining encounters for health care workers, and more than 256 million prevention outreach encounters.

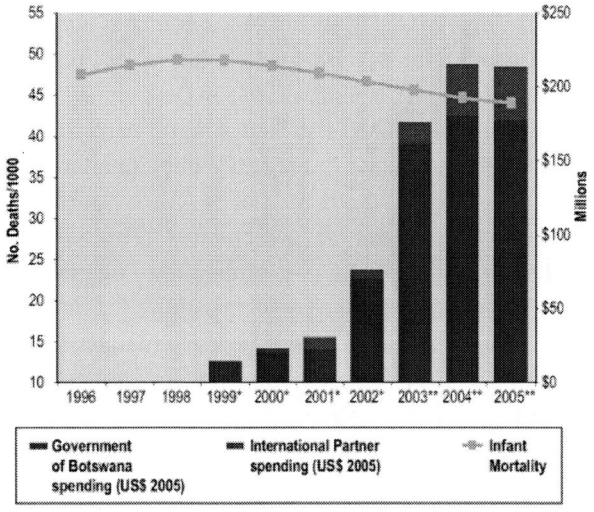

Infant mortality data provided by U.S. Census Bureau. Funding data is estimated based on data provided by the Government of Botswana and CDC; may not include all funding sources.

Figure 1. Infant Mortality and HIV Spending in Botswana.

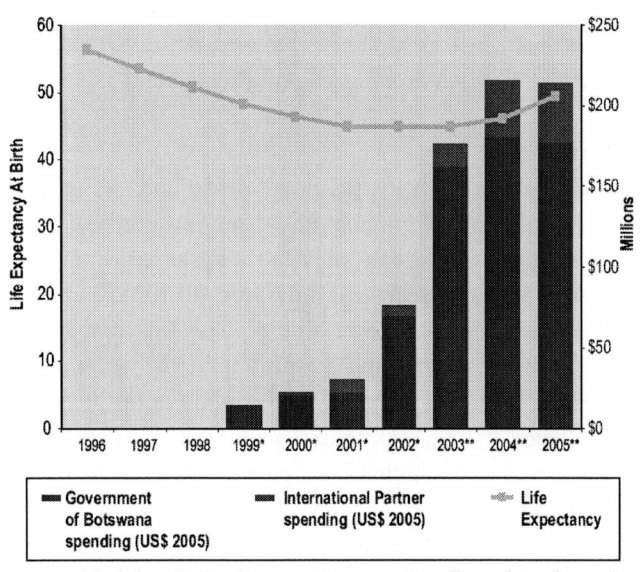

Life expectancy data provided by U.S. Census Bureau. Funding data is estimated based on data provided by the Government of Botswana and CDC; may not include all funding sources.

Figure 2. Life Expectancy and Spending in Botswana.

In addition to achieving Congressionally-mandated targets, the program has also had far-reaching health impacts in countries. A May 2009 study published in the *Annals of Internal Medicine* found that HIV-related mortality had dropped by 10.5% in 12 PEPFAR focus countries analyzed by researchers – implying that about 1.2 million deaths were averted due to the work of PEPFAR.[5] Studies presented at a July 2009 International AIDS Society conference illustrated that investments in fighting HIV/AIDS, including those of PEPFAR, contributed to population-level reductions in child and infant mortality.[6] For example, in Eastern Uganda, the increase in HIV/AIDS services is associated with a 83% reduction in non HIV-related infant mortality.[7] In addition, Botswana experienced declines in infant mortality and increases in life expectancy as HIV spending rose in the country.[8]

Beyond these contributions, PEPFAR also had a significant impact on the way health-related foreign assistance is delivered. Its interagency implementation model is overseen at the headquarters level by the Office of the U.S. Global AIDS Coordinator at the Department of State, and by the U.S. Ambassador at the country level. Through this interagency collaboration, PEPFAR has drawn upon the core strengths of agencies from across the USG to embody sound public health and development principles in its programming. PEPFAR integrates HIV prevention, treatment, and care services in a manner that supports an inclusive, multisectoral response. Its work draws upon the knowledge, access, and talents of local community- and faith-based organizations. The program leverages other development initiatives, including those in nutrition, education, and economic development, to maximize the overall impact of USG investments in HIV programming.

From its beginning, PEPFAR has demonstrated the clear role and impact of USG HIV/AIDS investments upon the larger global health arena. Prior to PEPFAR, many had given up on low-resource settings in the developing world as places where HIV infection was untreatable. The program has been successful in delivering HIV services, and created a new cadre of experts among local health care providers. The systems of care established and strengthened by PEPFAR can serve as a platform to expand, integrate, and co-locate primary and specialty care services to best serve the needs of infected and affected populations.

Challenges and Opportunities

Due to the investments through PEPFAR, the Global Fund to Fight AIDS, Tuberculosis, and Malaria and other stakeholders, much has been accomplished. HIV is no longer overwhelming the day-to-day operations of health systems in many heavily burdened countries. Because of these very successes, however, PEPFAR can and must do more. PEPFAR is evaluating its response to inform a next phase that emphasizes country capacity and sustainable responses while continuing support for existing and emerging prevention, care and treatment needs. PEPFAR's second phase builds upon its strengths and addresses some of the challenges faced by the program. This strategy examines how to best achieve PEPFAR's enormous potential as a health, development, and diplomatic tool.

Given the magnitude of the challenge faced at its creation, PEPFAR's initial emergency approach was critically needed, but had both positive and negative impacts on country-level health systems and budgets. At the beginning of the program, a focus on establishing services took precedence over prolonged engagement in planning and coordination with some country governments or other donors. At times, implementation did not fully complement existing national structures or plans. While the program has been applauded for its focus on service delivery targets, in some countries, this focus did not fully translate to a broader service delivery impact across the health sector. Access to quality services for all health conditions remains problematic in some areas. Given the innovative nature of many of PEPFAR's activities, there remains a need for a broad evaluation of program effectiveness and long-term impact.

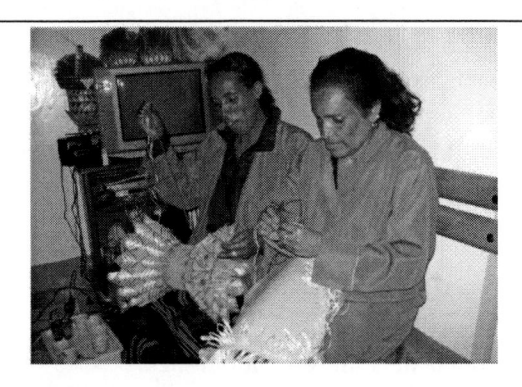

Through the PEPFAR-supported Mothers to Mothers (M2M) program at Bella Hospital in Ethiopia, mothers living with HIV/ AIDS provide advice to pregnant women about prevention of mother-to-child transmission services. Through the M2M program, mentor mothers such as Merima Abrar and Messelu Ketema, pictured above, bravely share their life experiences with pregnant women, counsel those who have just learned their HIV status, encourage them to live positively, and ensure they take their antiretroviral drugs regularly. Despite the challenges of this work, the program provides mentor mothers with the skills and confidence to teach their neighbors, and the ability to support their families economically through income generating activities. Merima and Messelu agree that the best reward of all is to see the birth of a child who is free of HIV.

PEPFAR places a premium on programming that responds to the country-level epidemic, but has faced challenges in achieving this goal. Responding to the country-level epidemic requires cooperation with other implementers and stakeholders. Barriers have sometimes existed to coordinating and providing technical assistance to Global Fund-financed programs at the country level. PEPFAR is strengthening multilateral collaboration and cooperation, and more fully incorporating high-level principles of the Paris Declaration. These include donor support of partner-country leadership and shared accountability for results. Such goals are a central aspect of PEPFAR's new Partnership Framework process, which promotes a more sustainable approach to the fight against AIDS at the country level.

While the interagency process has been one of PEPFAR's strengths, there has been some degree of interagency conflict at both country and headquarters level. PEPFAR was launched as a new way of doing business, causing some uncertainty among health and development experts who were unclear about their role in the new model. Field perspective and input have not always been reflected in policy or planning decisions. PEPFAR's extensive reporting requirements were not always harmonized with other USG development programs or other international indicators. Partner governments and country teams appropriately raised concerns about the impact of reporting requirements on field programming. Finally, the program has represented a significant scale-up of resources at Embassies without always having the commensurate increase in staff.

Increased investments in various disease- and issue- specific programs over the past decade have resulted in immense gains. There has been expanded interest in strengthening health systems as a way to reduce illness and death, particularly maternal mortality and childhood infectious diseases. PEPFAR now has the opportunity to strategically plan programs with greater consideration for the larger health systems impact. PEPFAR holds great potential for better across-the-board integration with broader health systems and development assistance, such as food, nutrition, and economic strengthening activities. Integration can contribute to larger goals involving infrastructure, governance, sustainability, and community- level health impacts, and allows PEPFAR to leverage its impact within a larger development context. In particular, the Global Health Initiative affords an opportunity to support expanded integration of PEPFAR programming with other USG health and development programming.

There is now a track record of success for bilateral initiatives like PEPFAR, multilateral funding vehicles like the Global Fund, and private donors like the Gates Foundation. Rather than emphasizing separate donor identities, opportunities exist to integrate, collaborate, and coordinate to support country-owned, country-guided programs. PEPFAR is working to evaluate existing data to replicate best practices, determine areas of efficiency, and support countries in a coordinated scale-up of proven and promising interventions. Learning from these successes is particularly important as the USG begins to consider larger foreign assistance reform. Lessons from PEPFAR can help to create systems that allow both PEPFAR and other health programs to be better integrated with all types of foreign assistance.

Investments in PEPFAR and the global AIDS fight overall, were and continue to be necessary. Six years after the creation of PEPFAR, AIDS is still a leading cause of death in many countries, and a continued threat around the world. 33.4 million people are living with HIV worldwide, and approximately 2.7 million new infections occurred in 2008.[9] For every two people who start treatment, five more are infected.[10] There still remain millions of children who have been orphaned by AIDS. Women and girls continue to face disproportionate impact of new infections, and WHO reports that AIDS is the leading cause of death worldwide for women in their reproductive years (ages 15-44).[11] Most-at-risk populations – including men who have sex with men (MSM), sex workers, and injecting drug users – continue to face stigma that limit their ability to obtain services, contributing to the wider transmission of HIV. The AIDS crisis is far from over. It will not end during the five year period covered by this strategy. Rather, the world will continue to struggle with continued need for prevention, care and treatment services – need which can only be addressed through a truly global response to the AIDS crisis.

PEPFAR has clearly proven that partnerships between the U.S. government and communities can provide comprehensive prevention, care, and treatment on a wide scale in low-resource countries. The program can now intensify collaboration with partner country governments and establish the conditions necessary to maintain these programs in both rural and urban areas. This strategy is designed to facilitate long-term sustainability and allow partner countries (formerly called "host countries") to lead their national and regional HIV/AIDS responses.

PEPFAR's Strategy

PEPFAR's Vision

In order to turn the tide of this global pandemic, PEPFAR will work through partner governments to support a sustainable, integrated, and country-led response to HIV/AIDS.

PEPFAR's Goals

Over the next five years, PEPFAR will work to achieve these five overarching goals:

1. Transition from an emergency response to promotion of sustainable country programs.
2. Strengthen partner government capacity to lead the response to this epidemic and other health demands.
3. Expand prevention, care, and treatment in concentrated and generalized epidemics.
4. Integrate and coordinate HIV/AIDS programs with broader global health and development programs to maximize impact on health systems.
5. Invest in innovation and operations research to evaluate impact, improve service delivery and maximize outcomes.

Key Concepts

As PEPFAR works in its next phase to achieve its goals and targets, it will be guided by the following key concepts. PEPFAR is working with its country teams to identify the best ways to implement these concepts as appropriate at the country level.

PEPFAR supports true partnerships with governments, in order to assist them as they lead and guide the response to their epidemics.

President Obama and Secretary Clinton have spoken of the need to work with governments in Africa and around the world to support good governance and leadership. The AIDS epidemic represents a shared global burden among nations, and PEPFAR represents an opportunity for the United States to support partner countries in assuming leadership of the response to their epidemics.

In the first five years of the program, PEPFAR focused on establishing and scaling up prevention, care and treatment programs. In some cases, it established programs and services outside of existing, often limited, health care delivery systems. Over this next phase, PEPFAR is focusing on transitioning from an emergency response to a sustainable one. It is working through bilateral, regional, and multilateral channels to improve and expand partner country capacity, enabling them to implement and manage a holistic response to the epidemic within the context of broader health sector concerns. PEPFAR's major goal is to enable governments to manage and coordinate quality health service delivery across all geographic regions within a country.

PEPFAR's role is to support partner government leadership to organize, develop, and coalesce donors and multilateral agencies around country-driven, country- responsive plans for the epidemic. Prevention, care and treatment activities are being supported with a focus on strengthening health systems and building sustainable partner country capacity. PEPFAR is expanding technical assistance and mentoring with country governments. Doing so supports a capable cadre of government professionals who can carry out the tasks necessary for a functioning health system, including financing and governance. The program is also facilitating partnerships between governments and a strong civil society, to ensure that citizens can work to provide support to and demand accountability from governments. Finally, the program is working to foster stronger regional collaboration and South-to-South technical assistance.

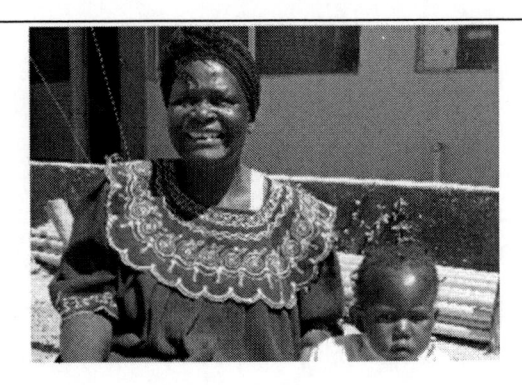

Two-year old Chipo is learning to walk, which is remarkable given the challenges of her early life. Chipo's mother passed away a month after her birth, and Chipo was diagnosed with HIV in addition to severe malnutrition, and was constantly sick. Chipo was cared for by her grandmother who lives in the remote village of Chitanda in Zambia's Central Province. To get Chipo the care she needed, they had to travel 82 kilometers to the nearest hospital because the Rural Health Center had no medication. In April 2008, mobile antiretroviral therapy (ART) outreach began at nearby Chitanda Rural Health Center and Chipo started obtaining treatment in her community. PEPFAR-supported mobile ART outreach currently covers seven remote locations across Central Province. As the mobile ART team provides services, they also train local health center staff. Over time, program responsibility will shift to the health center, freeing the mobile team to expand services to new locations.

In many of the countries where PEPFAR works, full transition of operations to partner country ownership and increased financing will take longer than five years to accomplish, but steps are being taken now to create the capacity for sustainability.

PEPFAR is expanding its emphasis on HIV prevention, and matching interventions and investments with epidemiological trends and needs in order to improve impact.

Prevention remains the paramount challenge of the HIV epidemic. While advances in treatment have revolutionized our response to AIDS, truly halting and reversing this epidemic will require a comprehensive, multisectoral prevention, care and treatment response.

There is no single population level intervention that can prevent HIV infection. A successful prevention program requires a combination of mutually reinforcing, continually evaluated interventions that are tailored to the needs and risks of different target populations. Since the beginning of the program, PEPFAR has worked to ensure that its interventions meet the need that exists in countries. Given that the epidemic is not static, changes within countries and regions – including the beneficial impact of prevention efforts – require a prevention response that identifies and deploys interventions to meet these new conditions.

This next phase of PEPFAR presents the opportunity to support countries in reassessing prevention portfolios in order to ensure that they are targeted for maximum impact. The major priority for PEPFAR's prevention programs in the short term is to support countries in mapping and documenting prevention needs. Doing so ensures that interventions are aligned to existing and emerging situations.

By working with countries to identify current drivers, including epidemics among subpopulations that may not be reached by general behavioral prevention messages, PEPFAR can target investments to greatest needs. PEPFAR is also expanding investments into high-impact prevention interventions, such as prevention of mother to-child transmission (PMTCT), male circumcision (MC), and services for injecting drug users. Finally, the program is working to identify, implement, and evaluate promising and innovative prevention methods, to expand our existing toolkit of interventions and advance the science around HIV prevention.

PEPFAR is committed to expanding access to high- quality prevention, care and treatment and immediate health needs while laying the groundwork for future sustainability.

In recognition of the integrated nature of prevention, care and treatment in PEPFAR, the USG continues to support a portfolio of activities tailored to the country context. PEPFAR is working with countries to ensure an appropriate balance among prevention, care and treatment activities. All of these activities are routinely monitored and evaluated in order to ensure that they are of high quality. They are also being analyzed to identify efficiencies and opportunities for integration with broader health and development efforts. PEPFAR targets its evidence-based prevention activities to the specific drivers of the epidemic, and supports pilots of new and innovative prevention programming.

In its care programming, PEPFAR works with countries to support a quality, integrated package of basic care and support interventions for people living with HIV and their caregivers. It also meets the care and support needs of OVCs. In the area of treatment, PEPFAR is working with partner countries to continue scale up, with a focus on specific populations.

PEPFAR's prevention, care and treatment activities are planned with consideration of how they may impact the overall health system, particularly human resources for health. To the extent possible, PEPFAR will incorporate mentoring and increased technical assistance into its programming. Doing so supports development of a cadre of partner country personnel – clinical, community-based, and civil service employees – with the skills to plan, finance, and operate these programs.

PEPFAR is responsive to people, not just to a virus.

Individuals who are infected and affected by HIV/AIDS experience the epidemic along with the other realities of their lives. PEPFAR activities must be responsive to the breadth of needs experienced by people living with HIV/AIDS, their families, and the communities hardest hit by the epidemic. High-quality prevention, care, and treatment activities will be implemented with consideration for their overall health systems impact. In addition, PLWHA are a critical part of the response, and must be involved in planning and implementation.

All PEPFAR programs – prevention, care, treatment, and linkages to larger health care services – must be evidence- based and driven by the needs of the people impacted by this epidemic. As a component of the Global Health Initiative, PEPFAR is working to implement women- centered care, and to ensure that its services are gender- equitable. Its programs address the particular vulnerabilities faced by women and girls, especially those who are impacted by gender-based violence. In order to make it easier for people with HIV to access all types of care they need, PEPFAR increases access to high-quality, low-cost care and treatment services. These services are responsive to the public health needs of marginalized communities, including injecting drug users, persons in prostitution, and men who have sex with men. PEPFAR also utilizes its services as a mechanism through which to advance the rights of populations that face stigma, and expand equal access to care.

PEPFAR is also expanding capability of existing service sites by linking HIV/AIDS services to other health interventions, rather than establishing and maintaining parallel systems of care. Given the larger structural barriers that exist in implementing effective HIV programming, PEPFAR is integrating services to respond to the nutrition, education, and economic development needs of AIDS-impacted communities.

In order to maximize U.S. investments, PEPFAR supports integration with other U.S. government programs in health and broader development sectors.

The success of PEPFAR is unambiguously linked to development mechanisms that expand the reach of bilateral HIV/AIDS assistance, promote country ownership, and increase sustainability of national health programs. PEPFAR is improving its own effectiveness by expanding efficiencies, engaging in joint programming, and working to transition programs to countries in both management and financial contexts. Over this second phase, PEPFAR is increasing efforts to integrate HIV services with existing country, USG-sponsored, and multilateral-financed programs. It is engaging in greater wraparound and joint programming with larger development initiatives, including the Global Hunger and Food Security Initiative, education, economic development, and legal and political reform. Doing so helps to create the structural changes that reduce risks for HIV transmission and expand access to quality care and support. This strategic integration also results in broader impact for both PEPFAR and the programs which it is leveraging.

PEPFAR has strong and robust engagement with multilateral partners and other external partners.

The challenges posed by the global AIDS crisis must be addressed as part of a shared global responsibility. PEPFAR is engaging in enhanced coordination with multilateral, regional, and bilateral partners, ensuring that USG efforts are not duplicative, and that donors are truly sharing the burden of the epidemic. In an affirmation of high level principles of the Paris Declaration, PEPFAR is working with its multilateral and bilateral partners to harmonize and align responses and support countries in achieving their nationally-defined HIV/AIDS goals.

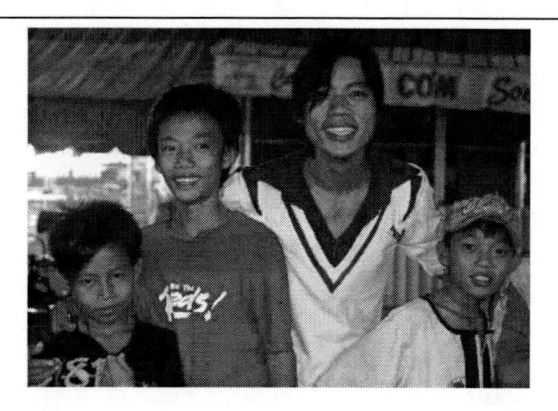

Like many street youth in Vietnam, 20 year old Sang has led a difficult life. For several years, he lived in a city park and spent his days stealing to support himself. He was the leader of a street youth gang that frequently fought with rival groups. Sang and his friends are among thousands of children and youth who live and work on the streets of Ho Chi Minh City. Life changed for Sang when a friend invited him to participate in Project N.A.M, a PEPFAR-supported peer education group. With training and support from the project's adult mentors, Sang and 20 others now work as HIV prevention peer educators. The project supports them to use a gender-based approach to help young men reduce risky sexual and drug use practices. The gender-based approach is two-fold: first, it promotes HIV prevention among young men themselves by helping them to reflect on and challenge gender norms that put young men, and consequently their partners, at risk. Second, it asks young men to question gender inequities. Sang has gained confidence and a sense of purpose: "As a peer educator, I know I'm a positive role model to other street youth and that I can help them make healthier decisions in their lives," he says.

PEPFAR is expanding involvement with the Global Fund, UNAIDS, World Health Organization, and other mechanisms. Doing so supports international consensus and action, progress toward joint programming and harmonized processes, and achievement of global goals such as reduction of commodity prices. PEPFAR also engages with foundations, public-private partnerships, regional bodies, and other civil society donors. Such collaboration supports partner country efforts to utilize all possible partners in developing a national response to HIV and to maximize the effectiveness of all funding streams. PEPFAR's overarching goal is to ensure that the actions of the donor community support efforts to enable countries to lead the response to their epidemics.

PEPFAR supports accountability, monitoring and evaluation, and implementation of efficiencies and best practices.

PEPFAR is committed to clear and transparent reporting of investments and results to ensure that its programs are accountable to taxpayers. PEPFAR works with independent auditors, including agency Inspectors General and the Government Accountability Office, and independent nongovernmental organizations to identify areas for improvement. Its next phase represents the opportunity to improve reporting mechanisms, data use, and monitoring and evaluation to maximize impact and investments. Now that PEPFAR has achieved success in prevention, care and treatment, programs are being reviewed for efficiencies to determine where more can be achieved with existing resources.

PEPFAR is objectively identifying best practices in quality service delivery, and looking for opportunities to replicate and establish cost-effective programs tailored to the country context. In addition, PEPFAR supports innovation, piloting new interventions to establish and expand the evidence base. The program is working to create greater transparency with its data, in order to facilitate identification of best practices and trends in PEPFAR that can contribute to larger systematic knowledge. PEPFAR is not a research initiative, but is expanding its current partnerships with implementers, researchers, and academic organizations to improve the science that guides this work. In keeping with the goal of sustainability, PEPFAR also supports the enhancement of local capacity to carry out monitoring and evaluation activities.

PEPFAR supports greater involvement of USG country teams and a strong interagency model.

PEPFAR has worked to decentralize programming and ensure that decisions on country-level activities are made by the USG country teams that are leading the ground- level response to the epidemic. For the past five years, these country teams have worked to rapidly expand and ensure quality health and social service delivery, while facing heavy reporting requirements. PEPFAR's interagency country teams ensure that programs meet the needs of the countries and communities where they work. PEPFAR is working to further integrate the field perspective into its policy and communications and reduce the reporting burdens and paperwork requirements placed on the field. Over the next few months, PEPFAR will be working closely with country teams to assist them in identifying the ways to best translate and implement these key concepts at the country level.

In order to enable USG country teams to respond to the best of their ability, PEPFAR continues to stress the importance of its interagency model. As a "whole of government" program, PEPFAR has coordinated efforts from multiple agencies to respond to global HIV. It is expanding coordination and linkages with broader USG health and development efforts as part of the Global Health Initiative. PEPFAR is assessing its innovative approaches to determine what elements contributed to interagency success at both the field and headquarters level, in order to replicate these more broadly. PEPFAR is also working to emphasize the core competencies of each agency. By achieving better coordination and building upon the strengths of USG personnel, PEPFAR can maximize its country-level impact.

ACRONYMS AND ABBREVIATIONS

ARV	Antiretroviral Drug
FY	Fiscal Year
IDU	Injecting Drug Users
Global Fund	Global Fund to Fight AIDS, Tuberculosis, and Malaria
MC	Male Circumcision
MSM	Men Who Have Sex with Men **OVC** Orphans and Vulnerable Children

PEPFAR	U.S. President's Emergency Plan for AIDS Relief
PLWHA	People Living with HIV/AIDS
PMTCT	Prevention of Mother-to-Child HIV transmission
UNAIDS	Joint United Nations Programme on HIV/AIDS
USG	United States Government
WHO	World Health Organization

End Notes

[1] http://whqlibdoc.who.int/publications/2009/9789241563857_eng.pdf, p 40

[2] http://data.unaids.org/pub/GlobalReport/2008/jc1510_2008 global report pp29 62_en.pdf

[3] http://www.unicef.org/publications/files/cob_layout6-013.pdf, p 3

[4] http://www.who.int/hiv/pub/tuapr_2009_en.pdf, p 5

[5] http://www.annals.org/cgi/content/full/0000605-200905190-00117v1

[6] http://www.iasociety.org/Web/WebContent/File/Leveraging%20HIV%20Investments% 20for%20Health%20Wome n%20and%20Kids%20%2822%20July%20FINAL%29.pdf

[7] Ibid.

[8] http://www.pepfar.gov/documents/organization/113827.pdf, p 10-11

[9] http://data.unaids.org/pub/Report/2009/2009_epidemic p. 6

[10] http://www.unaids.org/en/CountryResponses/UniversalAccess/default.asp

[11] http://whqlibdoc.who.int/publications/2009/978924 1 563857_eng.pdf, p 40

In: Global HIV/AIDS Threat and the U.S. Response
Editor: David R. Carmody
ISBN: 978-1-61324-568-2
© 2011 Nova Science Publishers, Inc.

Chapter 3

THE U.S. PRESIDENT'S EMERGENCY PLAN FOR AIDS RELIEF (FIVE-YEAR STRATEGY): ANNEX-PEPFAR AND PREVENTION, CARE AND TREATMENT

David R. Carmody

PREVENTION

Key Points

- A major short-term priority for PEPFAR's prevention programs is to support countries in mapping and documenting current and emerging prevention needs.
- PEPFAR's prevention programs will focus on scaling up high-impact, evidence-based, combination prevention approaches.
- Mutually reinforcing prevention interventions must be targeted to address needs of subpopulations in which new infections are concentrated.
- PEPFAR is supporting and evaluating promising and innovative practices to determine the effectiveness and impact of such interventions at both the country and global level.
- Linking treatment and care programs to prevention messaging allows PEPFAR to maximize its impact in all areas, particularly in reaching partners and families of people living with HIV/AIDS (PLWHA).
- Structural factors, such as existing economic, social, legal and cultural conditions contribute to increased risk for HIV infection. PEPFAR's prevention activities are addressing and evaluating the response to these factors.
- PEPFAR's prevention efforts will contribute to the global evidence base around prevention.
- PEPFAR is utilizing prevention of mother-tochild transmission (PMTCT) as a mechanism to both prevent transmission of HIV to children and support expanded access to care and related services for pregnant women.

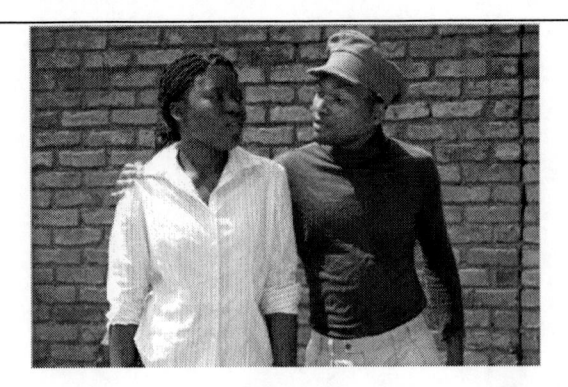

In Malawi, the PEPFAR-supported Lions Drama Group uses theatrical performances to educate audiences about HIV prevention and encourage behaviorchange. Thlupego Chisiza, founder of the Lions Group, knows his group's performances are creating impact. After performing in southern Malawi, a local businesswoman confided in him that seeing her life experience acted out in her community prompted her to take action and start actively encouraging young people to employ safe sexual practices.

Prevention remains the paramount challenge of the HIV epidemic, and preventing new infections represents the only long-term, sustainable way to turn the tide against HIV/AIDS. For any given population, the public health response must strike a balance between prevention opportunities and treatment needs. A successful prevention program requires a combination of mutually reinforcing interventions tailored to the needs of different target populations.

According to the Joint United Nations Programme on HIV/AIDS (UNAIDS), there were approximately 2.7 million new HIV infections in 2008, and 33.4 million people living with HIV.[1] New infections still far outpace the world's ability to add people to treatment. For every two people put on antiretroviral drugs (ARVs), another five become newly infected.[2] In recent years, several low- prevalence countries have had some success in containing their epidemics, concentrated in most-at-risk populations (MARPs). However, only a few high-prevalence countries have significantly reduced HIV prevalence. Increased attention is critical for hyperendemic countries, while simultaneously continuing to respond to countries with both concentrated and generalized epidemics.

CHALLENGES TO SUCCESSFUL PREVENTION PROGRAMS

Challenges in carrying out successful prevention programs encompass multiple factors, such as:

Lack of Country-level and Locally-specific Data

PEPFAR's prevention response is based upon HIV demographic and epidemiologic data. In many countries, there is a need for additional or updated data necessary to track the most recent new infections – primarily new infections over the past year. These data allow for outreach to the populations in which these infections are occurring. Without such ongoing surveillance, countries are unable to match timely investments to existing and evolving needs.

Existence of Multiple Epidemics and Need for Multiple Targeted Interventions

There is not a single HIV epidemic within any given country. Rather, multiple epidemics exist within diverse populations and social networks, including concentrated epidemics within larger generalized epidemics. Identifying and targeting interventions to match the needs of multiple populations is difficult, especially when such epidemics involve groups that are often marginalized and discriminated against. Stigmatized populations are frequently hidden and hard to reach with services. Effectively addressing a country's HIV epidemic must involve mutually- reinforcing interventions targeted to populations based upon epidemiological and demographic data. Specific populations, such as youth, women, transient populations, men who have sex with men (MSM), sex workers, and injecting drug users (IDUs), require programming tailored to their situation within the country context, rather than broad-based, national-level, generalized prevention messaging.

Need for Expanded Evaluation, Operations Research and Metrics

There are a number of evidence-based interventions used by PEPFAR and other HIV prevention programs. Several programs targeting most-at-risk populations have been proven to be effective. Certain interventions utilized in generalized epidemics, such as prevention of mother-to-child transmission and male circumcision (MC) also have a strong evidence base. More operations research regarding prevention is needed, particularly around general population prevention programs in high-prevalence countries. Although many small pilot programs involving behavior change interventions have proven effective, there is a need to demonstrate continued efficacy following scale-up of these pilots. At the global level, there is a need for additional research to better measure the impact of prevention programs and refine estimates of infections averted.

Stigma and Discrimination

The majority of HIV infections occur through sexual contact. In addition to sexual transmission, a significant number of infections occur due to sharing of needles, often in the context of injecting drug use. Stigma and discrimination create barriers to accessing key populations with critical prevention interventions. Denial about the epidemic can also contribute to perceptions of low risk and reduce demand for services. Finally, cultural and social norms may lead to policies that reinforce stigma and discrimination.

Structural Conditions

Existing economic, social, legal and cultural conditions often increase the risk of HIV transmission for individuals. For example, if a community treats sexual violence as a cultural norm, rather than a criminal act, those impacted by this violence may be unable to protect themselves from HIV or receive necessary care following the assault. Prevention must take into account the factors existing outside the health sector that impact risk and vulnerability to HIV. There is also a need for increased research and evaluation into the impact of structurally-based prevention interventions.

Inability to Capitalize on all Opportunities for Prevention

Multiple opportunities to advance prevention messaging are present in individual interactions with the healthcare system. There are also opportunities to reach existing audiences through social networks, schools, or mass media. With multiple demands on health, education, and social welfare systems, it is difficult to effectively utilize every opportunity to engage in prevention messaging.

Lack of Unified Messaging

In order for prevention messages to be effective, population-specific messages delivered by mass media, community mobilization activities, and interpersonal communication activities must be coordinated and mutually reinforcing. Otherwise, mixed messages and inconsistent information can dilute the impact of prevention programs.

Over the next phase, PEPFAR's prevention response will be guided by the following concepts:

- Supporting countries in reassessing their prevention response through mapping the epidemic, identifying the populations most impacted by new infections, and updating prevention strategies based upon these data;
- Assisting countries in implementing a combination of behavioral, biomedical, and structural interventions;
- Implementing, scaling up, and measuring the impact of proven and promising interventions, tools, and methodologies;
- Working with countries to target and reach most at-risk populations, no matter how stigmatized or marginalized these populations may be;
- Expanding the evidence base around prevention, through monitoring, evaluation, and operations research of prevention programming; and
- Contributing to international efforts to develop harmonized indicators and new surveillance methodologies.

Identifying Greatest Need: Mapping the Epidemic

A major short-term priority for PEPFAR's prevention programs is to support countries in mapping and documenting current and emerging prevention needs. This process includes surveillance, surveys and program mapping, and data analysis to craft and revise overall strategies to address the drivers of the epidemic. Through this mapping, PEPFAR can help governments develop and expand epidemiologically-driven responses, thus improving efforts to reduce overall HIV incidence.

For example, in Kenya, PEPFAR and the Ministry of Health conducted a revised Kenya AIDS Indicator Survey (KAIS). This survey was a tool designed to provide up-to- date information on HIV and other sexually transmitted infections (STIs). Following the data collection and analysis, PEPFAR and the Kenyan Government supported a series of HIV Prevention Summits. These Summits used findings from the KAIS that led to the development of a National HIV Prevention Strategy. With this National Prevention Strategy, PEPFAR has been able to ensure alignment with national priorities, improve coordination with other donors in accordance with a country plan, and increase efficiencies in the program. Over the next few years, PEPFAR will work to support the Kenyan government in implementing and assessing the impact of its prevention programming.

Priority Interventions

PEPFAR is working with countries to implement, monitor, and improve comprehensive HIV prevention programs targeted to specific populations in both concentrated and generalized epidemic settings. What follows below is additional detail regarding some of the interventions PEPFAR is at a national and local level. Given that prevention is not a static field, PEPFAR will evaluate implementation of additional activities as the science evolves.

COMBINATION PREVENTION

By combining quality biomedical, behavioral and structural interventions – known as "combination prevention" – countries can work over time in given geographic areas to craft a comprehensive prevention response. Components of combination prevention include:

- *Biomedical interventions*, such as prevention of mother-to-child transmission, use medical approaches to block infection, decrease infectiousness, or reduce infection risk. The treatment or intervention often acts as the platform for a larger prevention message. For example, PEPFAR's male circumcision package not only provides the actual circumcision procedure, but includes a package of prevention interventions, including risk reduction counseling and outreach to the sexual partner of the man being circumcised.

- *Behavioral interventions* include a range of approaches that address key behavioral outcomes – including delay of sexual debut, partner reduction, mutual monogamy, and correct and consistent use of condoms. Approaches are geared to motivate positive behavioral change in individuals, couples, families, peer groups or networks, institutions, and communities. These science-based, culturally- and age-appropriate interventions promote sustained behavior change through different, mutually-reinforcing program components. For example, mass media, community mobilization and interpersonal communication efforts are used in concert to encourage individuals, families, and communities to adopt and maintain healthy behaviors and norms.

- *Structural interventions* acknowledge that an individual's behaviors are in part governed by social, cultural, political, and economic norms. These interventions aim to change the larger societal, political, and economic contexts which can contribute to vulnerability and risk. For example, gender-based violence (GBV) has been linked to increased risk for HIV. Structural interventions targeting this risk include legal and policy changes that criminalize gender-based violence and result in increased awareness, reporting, and enforcement of penalties for those who engage in gender-based violence.

Prevention of Mother-to-Child Transmission (PMTCT)

Mother-to-child transmission is a significant cause of new infections among pediatric populations. Many factors, including lack of access to routine and ongoing antenatal care, have limited progress around PMTCT. In keeping with the Global Health Initiative (GHI) focus on women- centered approaches, PEPFAR is utilizing PMTCT as a mechanism to both prevent transmission of HIV to children and support expanded access to care and related services for pregnant women. Through PMTCT services, women can learn their status, accessing essential care if positive, and receiving information on ways to protect themselves if negative.

PEPFAR is increasing investments in PMTCT to support countries in expanding access to screening and coverage. It is working to ensure that every partner country with a generalized epidemic has both 80% coverage of testing for pregnant women at the national level, and 85% coverage of antiretroviral drug prophylaxis and treatment, as indicated, of women found to be HIV-infected. PEPFAR is also working to expand access to PMTCT to at-risk populations in countries with concentrated epidemics. To help the children of these mothers, PEPFAR supports antiretroviral prophylaxis regimens and essential medical care for HIV-exposed infants. These expanded PMTCT efforts strengthen overall maternal and child health care.

Male Circumcision (MC)

UNAIDS and the World Health Organization (WHO) have issued normative guidance stating that male circumcision should be recognized as an additional important intervention to reduce the risk of heterosexually acquired HIV infection in men.[3] PEPFAR supports MC as a component of a comprehensive HIV prevention program in sub-Saharan Africa, and is working to scale up quality MC programs as feasible and appropriate to the country context. In its next phase, PEPFAR is transitioning to a two- pronged MC assistance approach. This approach would simultaneously support the immediate demand for MC and allow governments to develop policies and the necessary infrastructure for more sustained service delivery.

The comprehensive MC interventions supported by PEPFAR include not only the MC surgery, but risk reduction counseling, sexually transmitted infection treatment, and HIV testing and counseling.

Health, Dignity and Prevention Programs for PLWHA

A strong body of literature supports the effectiveness of prevention interventions for PLWHA in a variety of settings. PEPFAR's prevention strategy for PLWHA and their partners includes both behavioral and biomedical interventions in clinic and community-based settings. Examples of these behavioral interventions include correct and consistent use of condoms, disclosure of status to partners, partner and family testing, reduction in number of sexual partners, reduction of alcohol use, and adherence to HIV medications which decrease viral load. Examples of these biomedical interventions include management of STIs in PLWHA and their sex partners and services to reduce maternal-to-child-transmission of HIV. PEPFAR is working with partner governments to integrate these interventions as part of the standard package of care at care and treatment sites. Civil society organizations and community-based groups providing these services will be linked to this larger clinical network.

Behavior Change Communication (BCC)

Throughout sub-Saharan Africa, key drivers of the epidemic include: multiple and concurrent sexual partnerships (MCP); intergenerational and transactional sex; low rates of male circumcision and of correct and consistent condom use; high rates of STIs; and high levels of alcohol use. PEPFAR supports a diverse range of culturally- and age-appropriate and comprehensive behavior change programming targeted to the country context.

Behavior change programming should include:

- Mutually reinforcing activities, including a mix of mass media, community mobilization, small-group and individual interventions that reflect best practice in BCC; and
- Prevention messages that address key epidemic drivers, are based on formative research, and are coordinated and delivered across both community and clinical settings.

PEPFAR will support efforts to expand the evidence base around behavior change communication, enabling more effective programming for generalized epidemics. In addition, PEPFAR will work with countries to focus BCC not only on behavior change at the individual level, but culture-wide change that addresses the gender and social norms contributing to HIV infection.

Testing and Counseling

Each testing and counseling encounter is an important opportunity to reinforce and share prevention messaging. Expanding testing and counseling diminishes the stigma associated with knowing one's status. Individuals who test HIV-positive and who are exposed to strong behavior change interventions can reduce their risk of onward transmission. Individuals who test negative can receive counseling and information to help protect themselves and remain

HIV-free. PEPFAR is working to link testing and counseling with clinical and community interventions, and improve referrals to care, treatment, prevention, and necessary supportive services. It is also working with governments to implement public health interventions that allow past contacts of PLWHAs to get tested and receive necessary prevention and treatment services. For those that are HIV-negative but are participating in high-risk behaviors, PEPFAR will work to implement modified case management with sustained prevention interventions. Finally, PEPFAR is working with countries to expand the use of rapid test kits, in order to enable more widespread use of testing outside of health facilities.

Safe Blood and Injection Safety

Medical injections and blood draws are among the most common health care procedures worldwide. In developing countries, the risk of contracting HIV from a blood transfusion is magnified by weak health care infrastructures and inadequate supplies of safe blood. Women and children are at greatest risk, due to the frequent use of blood transfusions to treat complications during pregnancy, childhood anemia associated with malaria, and various trauma incidents. To date, PEPFAR has engaged in significant support for blood safety programs. It is supporting infrastructure and lab development, technical assistance and training, and universal testing of blood units for HIV and other transfusion-transmissible infections.

Safe medical injection practices protect not only patients, but also local community members and health care workers who are routinely exposed to needles and other medical sharps. PEPFAR is supporting countries to develop safe injection policies, purchase safe injection equipment and supplies, and expand safe disposal among health care workers and community members. In addition to promotion of universal precautions, PEPFAR will work to reduce demand for unnecessary injections and promote appropriate use of transfusions.

Innovation in Prevention

Over the next five years, research may demonstrate the efficacy of additional prevention interventions such as microbicides, pre-exposure prophylaxis, and vaccines. PEPFAR will remain involved in and supportive of partner country and international efforts to identify and implement successful prevention interventions.

Microbicides, an invisible, women-controlled prevention method, will be a great asset to prevention interventions when available. PEPFAR supports efforts to find a safe, effective microbicide that can be easily used in low-resource settings. It will continue to assist partner countries in preparations for eventual microbicide introduction, regulation, manufacturing, and distribution.

There is currently a great deal of research under way involving the preventive impacts of treatment, including studies regarding the protective effect of pre-exposure prophylaxis with antiretrovirals. If efficacy is shown, demonstration projects will be essential to determining the feasibility of this approach, resource requirements, and the potential for scale-up.

Research on vaccines continues to propel hopes that an HIV vaccine can be an important part of HIV prevention strategies in the future. Even a partially efficacious vaccine could have tremendous impact in HIV prevention when coupled with other interventions. It is important for PEPFAR to continue to have links to vaccine research, as well as efforts to determine where effective vaccines can have the greatest public health impact.

Strategic Populations

PEPFAR's prevention strategies must be responsive to the drivers of the epidemic and address the needs of most-at risk populations in both generalized and concentrated epidemics. Prevention messaging needs to educate populations about the way the virus is transmitted. Successful prevention interventions help individuals to acknowledge and identify risk factors in their lives and actions they can take to protect themselves. The following describes ways in which PEPFAR will support countries in implementing prevention programs for specific populations:

Vulnerable women and girls

Nearly 60% of HIV infections in sub-Saharan Africa occur among women.[4] PEPFAR is working through its gender strategy to address the needs of women and girls, many of whom are vulnerable due to structural conditions that limit their ability to access or utilize prevention programming. It is especially important for PEPFAR and countries to address the needs of girls and young women in relationships with older men, as these types of relationship are often common in hyperendemic areas. More detailed information about PEPFAR's work with women, girls, and gender activities can be found in additional annex documents available at *www.pepfar.gov/strategy/*.

Men who have sex with men (MSM)

Reaching MSM in both generalized and concentrated epidemic settings poses significant challenges. In several of the countries in which PEPFAR works, homosexual activity is defined as a criminal act, and may result in detention or arrest for those suspected of engaging in MSM activity. Governments are often reluctant to engage in outreach to these communities. Cultural mores and stigma may make MSM reluctant to disclose possible risks in a clinical setting. In addition, transgender populations face significant stigma and barriers to receiving appropriate health services. In order to address the health needs of these populations, PEPFAR is working with countries to engage in the following:

Identifying the need in the MSM community

Rates of HIV infection among MSM are often much higher than the general population. A major prevention priority for PEPFAR is helping governments to engage in the research necessary to map their epidemic and identify increased risk existing among subpopulations including MSM. This data-driven base makes it easier for public health programs to target prevention efforts.

Removing Stigma and Discrimination

PEPFAR will work to ensure that its prevention, care, and treatment programs are free from stigma and discrimination directed toward clients.

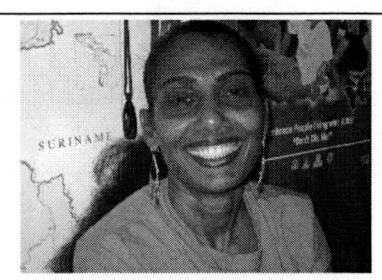

Evan – a former sex worker – is now educating peers about safer sexual practices and raising HIV/AIDS awareness through the PEPFAR-supported "Keep the Light On" project. The project is aimed increasing peer education of sex workers in Guyana to provide HIV/ AIDS education to their peers and to teach them safer sexual practices.

Supporting MSM access to prevention, care, and treatment

PEPFAR supports country government policies that ensure that MSM have equal access to health care, HIV/AIDS information and supportive services, and do not face arrest or detention for seeking these services.

Persons in Prostitution

Individuals who engage in or procure transactional sex, even on an occasional basis, are at higher risk for HIV. The intersection of trafficking in persons and prostitution further complicates efforts to provide needed HIV services. Prostitution is associated with psychological and physical risks, and PEPFAR is working with countries to help persons in prostitution get the prevention, care, and treatment services that they need. PEPFAR supports countries in the following activities:

Engaging in targeted prevention, care, and treatment outreach

PEPFAR is supporting efforts to provide basic HIV prevention, care, and treatment services to persons in prostitution. In many countries, cultural norms contribute to stigmatization of sex workers, limiting their ability to seek or obtain care. PEPFAR is working with governments to ensure that access to health care and social services is not denied because an individual is a sex worker.

Helping governments to support alternatives to prostitution

From a public health perspective, it is important not only to reduce the overall risk to individuals who are engaged in transactional sex, but to prevent people from turning to transactional sex in an economic crisis. PEPFAR is working with governments to support programs that increase educational and economic opportunity for sex workers, and that keep at-risk youth in schools or vocational training. It is also important to ensure that prevention programs and personnel recognize the risks associated with occasional transactional sex.

Working to reduce demand

Through its gender programming, PEPFAR is working with countries to change behavioral expectations that promote transactional sex as "masculine" behavior. It also works to ensure that men who procure sex take measures to protect themselves and all their sexual partners.

Injecting drug users

Comprehensive prevention packages for IDUs not only reduce immediate risks of transmission, but enable this population to receive care to treat and end their addiction. In multilateral fora, the Obama administration has supported a package of prevention to injecting drug users that mirrors the prevention package supported by the UNAIDS/United Nations Office on Drugs and Crime (UNODC)/WHO Technical Guide on harm reduction programs in relation to HIV.[5] The Technical Guide recommends that programs directed toward IDUs should include a comprehensive package of nine activities. PEPFAR is currently working with agencies across the U.S. Government (USG) to determine the best way forward in supporting this comprehensive package.

Youth

The categorization of "youth" is often misleading, as youth not only encompass multiple age ranges, but also face various types of risk. PEPFAR's programming for youth is medically accurate, age-appropriate, and targeted to needs based upon behavior. Behavioral interventions include delaying age of sexual debut, discouraging MCP or intergenerational sex, and providing information about consistent and correct use of condoms. PEPFAR will work with countries to strengthen school-based programs. HIV prevention messages that address the needs of both girls and boys will be integrated into life skills curricula. PEPFAR will also encourage governments to involve youth as part of the civil society response to the epidemic, so that policies targeting adolescents and young adults are realistic and responsive.

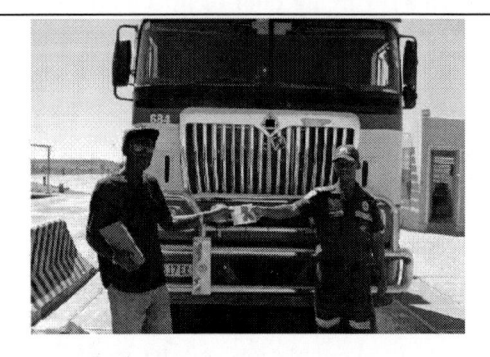

A Walvis Bay Corridor Group member hands a Namibian truck driver a copy of the NamibiAlive II CD. The CDs, which were produced by two Peace Corps Volunteers to raise awareness about HIV/AIDS, are given to truck drivers in an effort to educate and prevent the spread of HIV/AIDS among industry employees.

While much of the focus on youth involves BCC, it is important to recognize the diversity of situations faced by the youth PEPFAR serves. Youth exist among mostat-risk populations. Given the rates of child marriage in some PEPFAR countries, there are a significant number of girls and young women in marriages who need information about how to protect themselves from HIV infection. Confounding these prevention interventions are the gender inequities that may limit the power of young women in these relationships. Youth who are out of school present particular risks, as do orphans and vulnerable children (OVC). These populations may need prevention messaging that is packaged along with vocational or other social support programming to address their economic needs. PEPFAR is working with countries to ensure that youth programming – including OVC programming – is responsive to the needs of out-of school youth.

Mobile populations

Truck drivers, migrant workers, and the military all pose significant challenges for HIV prevention efforts. The transient natures of these populations often limit exposure to prevention messaging, and also may increase opportunities to engage in high-risk behavior. Involuntarily mobile populations, such as internally displaced persons or other refugees, can be at high risk for HIV, particularly due to increased risk of sexual assault. Given the fact that these populations are moving across borders, governments may be less aware of their needs. There is difficulty cataloging and documenting need among these rapidly changing communities. The cross-border nature of these populations and their related epidemics exemplifies the need for cross-border and regional programming for these vulnerable populations. PEPFAR is working with governments, regional institutions, and multilateral organizations to provide outreach to these populations and ensure that comprehensive services are accessible to them.

Incarcerated populations

Prevention work with incarcerated individuals affords an opportunity to diminish risk of transmission within and outside the correctional facility. Governments often do not place an emphasis on the ways in which a revolving door of prison populations can amplify risk in the general population. PEPFAR is supporting governments to minimize transmission within correctional facilities, educate and involve law enforcement in prevention activities, and ensure that adequate HIV prevention, care, and treatment services are available within prison settings.

Health Care Workers

To date, PEPFAR has supported post-exposure prophylaxis (PEP) treatment for health workers who suffer needle-stick injuries. PEPFAR is continuing to work with countries in developing a health care infrastructure that follows internationally-accepted infection control protocols. PEPFAR supports implementation of universal precautions, and increased availability of basic medical supplies to limit the risks faced by these workers.

MOVING FORWARD WITH PREVENTION

Years 1-2

- Support countries in efforts to collect data and map drivers of the multiple epidemics in a country.
- Assist countries to develop and implement short- and long-term combination prevention strategies linked to epidemiologic and demographic data.
- Scale up existing high-impact interventions, maximizing linkages to care, treatment and broader health services.

- Identify evidence-based best practices, engaging in piloting of promising interventions, and increase operations research for prevention programming.
- Begin impact evaluation of prevention programs and establish baselines for evaluations of new activities.
- Work with countries to target and reach most-atrisk populations, no matter how stigmatized or marginalized these populations may be.

Years 3-5

- Scale up innovative programs based on operations research, basic program evaluations and other prevention research from years 1-2.
- Engage in targeted remapping as necessary to ensure that prevention investments meet need.

STIGMA AND DISCRIMINATION

Using public health principles as a foundation, PEPFAR supports HIV prevention, care, and treat¬ment activities as a mechanism to advance the rights of people who are marginalized, stigmatized, dis¬criminated against, and denied access to essential care. Advances in expanding access to quality ser¬vices in low-resources settings have highlighted the discrimination that still exists.

It is difficult to quantify the impact of stigma and discrimination. There are no statistics to document the number of people denied access to care because of their HIV status, gender, or sexual orientation, or the number of people who choose not to go to a clinic because they face judgmental workers. However, anecdotal evidence exists. Stigma results in individuals not adhering to treatment because doing so will mean explaining to others exactly why they are taking medication. Fear of disclosure means that children stop receiving HIV services because their mothers can no longer pass off frequent clinic visits as routine pediatric monitoring. Such stories demonstrate why it is imperative for PEPFAR and its partner countries to provide impartial, science-based information, education, care and support services.

In order for PEPFAR to support countries in reducing stigma and discrimination, it will focus on the following activities over its next phase:

Emphasizing Support for Marginalized Populations as an Essential Part of Country Engagement

As PEPFAR moves towards increased country ownership, discussions with government are addressing the need for health and social service structures that are responsive to all people living with and at-risk for HIV. Doing so will require policies that address the drivers of the epidemic in country and provide equitable access to quality services for marginalized populations. By demonstrating the public health benefits that result when prevention, care, and treatment are provided to otherwise stigmatized communities, PEPFAR is emphasizing the importance of a comprehensive, inclusive response.

Elimination of "Double Stigma"

PEPFAR trainings, guidance, programming, and engagement with countries will be geared to help with the identification and targeting of "double stigma." This term refers to the stigma faced by people who are both HIV-positive and part of a marginalized population – for example, HIV-positive MSM, or HIV-positive IDUs. Quality care and treatment programs must be fully accessible to all subpopulations within the HIV-positive population. PEPFAR will work with the health care workers it supports to address the issues around adherence and retention in care that arise when people who are HIV-positive are unable to disclose their status in unsupportive communities.

Continued Support for Greater Involvement of PLWHA

Since the early years of the epidemic, a major component of the HIV movement has been meaningful involvement of persons living with HIV. As PEPFAR increases engagement with countries, it will emphasize this principle as one that should be incorporated in planning, prioritization and implementation of national HIV programs. Greater involvement of intended recipients of services enables programs to be culturally appropriate and configured for optimal effectiveness. PEPFAR and its country teams will also improve their efforts to involve PLWHA and their input in all aspects of its work.

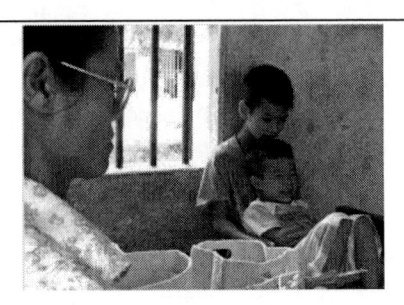

Kindergartener Binh Luom relaxes at home after school with his older brother and his mother. Thanks to the PEPFAR-supported Hanoi Legal Clinic, Binh and other HIV-positive children in Vietnam are able to attend school.

Continued Support for Greater Involvement of Persons from Most-at-risk Populations

PEPFAR will work to increase engagement with persons from most-at-risk or targeted populations in the planning and implementation of national HIV programs. Representatives from key populations should be included in all aspects of their programming.

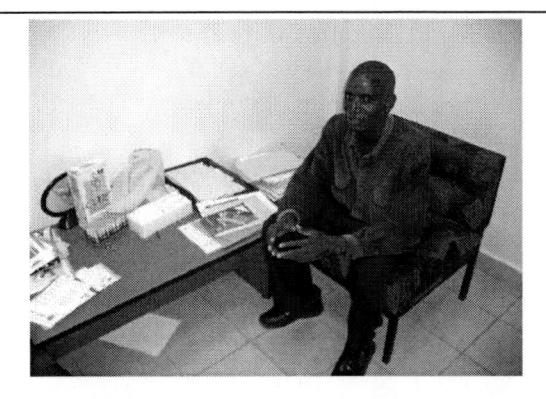

After learning that he is HIV-positive, Deodatus joined a post-test club where he was able to find support, discuss his feelings, access information on HIV prevention and treatment, and share experiences with other people living with HIV/AIDS in Tanzania. Deodatus then received training and obtained a job sharing his positive living experiences with other Tanzanians who are accessing HIV counseling and testing services.

CARE AND SUPPORT

Key Points

- PEPFAR is working with countries to develop strategies to reduce HIV-related morbidity and mortality.
- Care programs should increase early identification of PLWHA and expand referrals into comprehensive Health, Dignity and Prevention programs.
- PEPFAR is working with countries to expand coverage of a quality basic package of care and support services for PLWHA and their families.
- There needs to be clear linkages between care and support services in homes, communities, and clinical care facilities.
- PEPFAR is supporting countries in efforts to increase appropriate pain management and palliative care.
- Populations that are often marginalized and face discrimination must have equal access to quality care and support services.
- PEPFAR will expand monitoring and evaluation of diverse care and support services by working to increase impact evaluations and link quality of life gains to care services.
- Despite the reduction in HIV-related death rates in PEPFAR countries, there is a need for pain and symptom management and palliative care to assist PLWHA.
- PEPFAR is working to increase the numbers of home-based care and community health workers and support more strategic deployment of these workers by partner governments.

The medical needs of an HIV-positive individual begin long before initiation of ART. It is critical to identify HIV-infected persons early, refer them to services, and retain them in care. Many of the care and support services offered to HIV-infected persons can improve health and quality of life, and reduce HIV-related complications and mortality. These services are part of a continuum of care offered from the time of initial HIV diagnosis, prior to and during ART, and continuing through end-of-life care.

Care and support services provided by PEPFAR comprise a broad range of activities, exclusive of ARV treatment, that are available to HIV-infected and affected individuals. These activities, including clinical, psychological, social, spiritual and preventive services, seek to increase retention in care, maximize functional ability, and minimize morbidity. From 2004 to 2008, the number of sites providing care and support in the 15 original focus countries increased from 3,126 to over 13,000. Over this same time period, care was provided to more than 10.1 million people.

PEPFAR has developed a package of interventions with proven efficacy in both reducing HIV-associated morbidity and mortality and reducing HIV transmission. Implementing this package provides multiple opportunities to integrate and coordinate with other health and development activities. This basic preventive care package may differ depending on the setting and the prevalence of other HIV-associated infections, but often includes many of the following interventions:

- Prophylaxis for opportunistic infections – most importantly, cotrimoxazole, which has been shown to significantly reduce mortality in HIV-infected individuals;
- Screening, prophylaxis and treatment for tuberculosis;
- Improved screening and treatment of opportunistic infections;
- Increased access to safe drinking water and promotion of basic hygiene and sanitation;
- Provision of insecticide-treated bednets;
- Improved nutrition, including nutritional and micronutrient supplementation, which may reduce mortality independent of ART, and improve outcomes for patients on ART;
- Health, Dignity and Prevention Programming for PLWHA and their families; and
- Provision of HIV testing and counseling for family members and other contacts.

In addition, a number of other services may be offered under the "care and support" umbrella, such as:

- Prevention, diagnosis, and treatment for opportunistic infections and other HIV-associated complications;
- Palliative care, including management of pain and other symptoms;
- Screening and treatment for cervical cancer – an opportunistic infection – currently provided through pilot programs in a number of countries; and
- Economic strengthening and support activities, so that PLWHAs can continue to support themselves and their families.

In its next phase, PEPFAR will build upon its successes and emphasize following activities:

- Optimizing early identification, referral, and retention of HIV-infected individuals, so they have access to the interventions described above;
- Reducing HIV-related morbidity and mortality, utilizing the interventions described above;
- Working at the country level to expand coverage and access to a quality basic care package for PLWHAs, particularly through integration of care with other health and development programming; and
- Improving the quality of life for PLWHAs and their families, and measuring this improvement through periodic special surveys or other evaluation tools.

Pain Management and Palliative Care

Despite the reduction in HIV-related death rates in PEPFAR countries, there is a need for pain and symptom management and palliative care to assist PLWHA. Even with expanded coverage and access to care, AIDS is still a leading cause of death in many of the countries where PEPFAR works. In many countries, access to strong pain medications (e.g. opioids) is extremely limited, especially outside of hospital settings. The definition of palliative care varies based upon the country context; the term means "end of life" care to some, while others define it to mean all care provided subsequent to a diagnosis of HIV infection. Patient-centered palliative care can be implemented either in the home, or in a community- based or facility setting, like a hospice, but there is a strong need to ensure continuity of quality care.

Many countries have restrictive policy environments that reduce access to pain management. Pain assessment and management should be included as part of the basic package of care services for PLWHAs. PEPFAR will continue to support policy changes that ensure that pain management is included both in guidelines and actual clinical services for PLWHAs. In addition, PEPFAR has supported civil society groups in work with their governments to strengthen commodity systems, train providers, and expand access to opioids for pain management.

PEPFAR's palliative care programs help to alleviate the burden of caregiving for families, particularly for children and adolescents who may otherwise be forced to drop out of school to care for ill parents. These programs also help families deal with the impact of HIV upon their loved ones. PEPFAR is working with countries to improve linkages between home or hospice-based palliative care and comprehensive clinical services, particularly given the challenges in accessing trained palliative care providers.

Home-Based Care and Community Health Workers

A significant proportion of PEPFAR's basic care package, developed to support country-led strategies, involves interventions that can be provided outside of a clinical setting and be linked to larger development efforts. In rural areas and places where clinics are overcrowded, home-based care and community health workers provide essential services and strengthen the reach of a health system.

Home-based care is an important part of relieving the caregiving burden and providing extra support to families. However, home-based care is not a substitute for comprehensive clinical care, which is generally facility- based. There must be close oversight and clear linkages between clinical, home- and community-based care to ensure that HIV-infected individuals have access to a full range of clinical care services. Expansion of health center-level support and supervision must occur in concert with expansion of home-based care, in order to ensure adequate quality in both home and facility settings.

Prior to the need for end-of-life palliative care, the home is also an important staging area for messaging and care from community health workers. Through routine home visits, workers provide anticipatory guidance to PLWHA and their families and reinforce clinic-delivered messages. Community-based workers deliver components of the basic care package, like safe water kits and cotrimoxazole. It is essential for community health workers to be well- trained and linked to a clinic-based facility. PEPFAR is working to increase the numbers of home-based care and community health workers and support more strategic deployment of these workers by partner governments.

PEPFAR is also working to support countries in health systems strengthening efforts that encompass care and support. Such activities may include:

- Ensuring trained health care workers receive appropriate supervision, training and support in facility, community, and home-based care settings;
- Improving linkages and referrals between facility, community, and home-based care programs to reinforce quality provision of care; and
- Assuring reliable supplies of critical commodities.

Given the high level of decentralization that occurs in care programming, PEPFAR is working with countries to ensure that services are available to all PLWHAs and affected populations without discrimination. Efforts to improve quality should also result in standard protections for patients, so that no PLWHA will be deterred from seeking and receiving care. In addition, PLWHA communities need to be engaged in efforts to plan and implement care and support services.

MOVING FORWARD WITH CARE AND SUPPORT

Years 1-2

- Support countries in defining and monitoring delivery of a basic package of care for PLWHA and their families, based upon country-level epidemiology and demographic data.
- Help countries determine, map and develop plans to meet the need for care and support services, especially in rural and underserved areas.
- Work with countries to establish pain management policies.
- Support additional training and supportive supervision for community health workers to provide home- and community-based care.

- Scale up existing high-impact care interventions and conduct robust program monitoring.
- Identify promising and best practices.
- Work with PLWHA communities to develop an active dialogue with policy and planning bodies, in order to allow for constructive feedback on effectiveness and continuous improvement of services.

Years 3-5

- Engage in special surveys or other evaluation tools to determine impact of care activities on quality of life of PLWHA and their families.
- Continue to support additional training for community health workers to provide home-based and community-based care.
- Work to ensure that increases in access to care are accompanied by increases in quality of care.
- Expand promising practices and successful care pilot programs, such as those addressing cervical cancer needs for HIV-positive women.

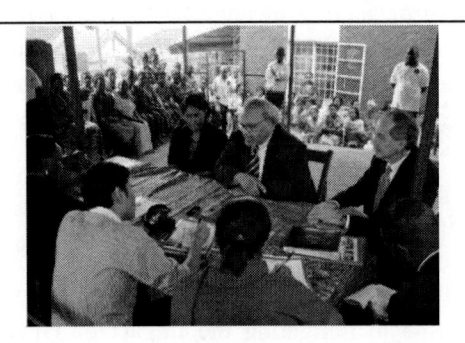

In Uganda, Ambassador Eric Goosby, U.S. Global AIDS Coordinator, participates in a press conference with Noelina Namukisa, Executive Director of Meeting Point, and Mike Strong, Uganda PEPFAR Coordinator. Meeting Point International, a Ugandan non-governmental organization, provides assistance to persons and families affected and infected with HIV/AIDS, with particular attention to orphans. The organization operates in four slums near Kampala, including one slum inhabited largely by those displaced by the civil war in the north.

ORPHANS AND VULNERABLE CHILDREN

Key Points

- PEPFAR's 10% earmark reflects the importance of the program's role in mitigating the impact of HIV/ AIDS for millions of children and adolescents living in affected communities.

- In order to ensure a true continuum of care, PEPFAR will assist countries to bridge the gaps between medical, social service, and civil society stakeholders, and coordinate support services with prevention, treatment and care programs.
- PEPFAR is working with partner governments to strengthen the capacity of families and communities to provide quality family-based care and support for OVC.
- PEPFAR-supported programming is age- appropriate, situation-specific, and cognizant of the multitude of needs among child and adolescent OVC in family or other situations.
- PEPFAR is working closely to integrate OVC programming with other USG efforts and multilateral efforts around education, food and nutrition, and livelihood assistance as part of a robust, comprehensive response to the needs of OVC.
- PEPFAR will increase efforts in youth livelihood development initiatives, focusing on higher levels of skill development.

According to the United Nations Children's Fund (UNICEF), approximately 15 million children worldwide have lost one or both parents to AIDS. Nearly 12 million of these children live in sub-Saharan Africa.[6] Many more children have been made vulnerable because of family illness and the widespread impact of HIV/AIDS on their communities. OVC populations will continue to grow as HIV incidence rates increase.

Although the vast majority of OVC can be found in family situations, some OVC live in institutions, in youth-headed households, or on the streets. The epidemic has decimated populations of teachers, healthcare workers, police, and other service providers that help to create strong networks of support for children and adolescents. As a result, OVC are more vulnerable to abuse and exploitation, and are also more likely to engage in unsafe behaviors, increasing the risk of HIV infection.

As part of the reauthorization of PEPFAR, Congress maintained the requirement to direct 10% of PEPFAR program funds be directed to OVC activities. This 10% earmark reflects the importance of PEPFAR's role in mitigating the impact of HIV/AIDS for the millions of children and adolescents living in affected communities.

PEPFAR is supporting child-centered, family-focused, community-based, and government-supported OVC programming. This evidence-based programming targets the full range of OVC needs at different developmental stages. It is linked with broader development efforts around education, food and nutrition, and livelihood assistance. PEPFAR works with countries to address the long-term impact of HIV/AIDS on child development. The quality services provided to OVC today can benefit the future well-being of a partner country. In its next phase, PEPFAR is supporting countries in pursuing the following objectives in OVC programming:

Building national systems of care

In an effort to promote a harmonized national response to the impact of HIV/AIDS on child development, PEPFAR is supporting and building capacity for multisectoral approaches. These efforts encourage governments to coordinate among various ministries, including those overseeing education, food and nutrition, social welfare, and health. PEPFAR is contributing to this coordination by ensuring that its OVC programs are integrated with other USG programs targeting children and vulnerable populations. In order to ensure a true continuum of care, PEPFAR will assist countries to bridge the gaps between medical, social service, and civil society stakeholders, and coordinate support services with prevention, treatment and care programs.

At the national level, PEPFAR is facilitating the adoption of child-friendly policies to address the needs of children infected and affected by HIV/AIDS, and to encourage alignment with broader health systems strengthening efforts. In keeping with PEPFAR's focus on creating government capacity for management and operation of HIV services, programs will also support the training of professional and paraprofessional staff. Finally, PEPFAR is supportive of country efforts to develop national standards for quality services provided by both the public and the private sector.

Strengthening the capacity of families and communities to care for vulnerable children

In Africa, an estimated 95% of orphaned children are cared for by other family members or neighbors.[7] Much of the current research on OVC care and support identifies family environments as better able to meet the needs of OVC than more institutional models. Many families caring for OVC are already impoverished and overextended. Children within these households often face great risk of malnutrition, disease, and limited access to education and health care. PEPFAR is working with governments to prioritize family-focused and community-based programs that strengthen the capacity of caregivers and communities to function as social safety nets. OVC programs should assess, monitor, and address, as needed, the well-being of OVC within six key areas: food and nutrition, shelter and care, protection, health, psychosocial, and education. Progress in these areas is measured across countries using the standardized Child Status Index (CSI) tool, developed to monitor PEPFAR's OVC programming.

Developing and targeting need-based OVC responses that are sensitive to the diversity of sub-populations within the larger OVC population

The needs of OVC vary according to age, gender, socioeconomic status, and geography. Various studies and research tools have recently contributed to the development of more effective and targeted strategies for specific sub-sets of the OVC population. PEPFAR is working with partner countries to ensure that the diverse needs of OVC are included in efforts to identify, map, and plan to address overall HIV/AIDS needs in a given country.

In its next phase, PEPFAR is also coordinating with other USG and donor efforts to expand country-led initiatives intended to identify and address the needs of several previously neglected sub-sets. For example:

- To better address the needs of newborns, infants, and toddlers, PEPFAR is strengthening linkages with food and nutrition programming, PMTCT and adult and pediatric treatment sites. It will also improve training for community health workers and home visitors to monitor child growth and development.
- To better address the needs of young school-age children, PEPFAR is linking programs to basic education initiatives, enabling OVC to stay in school.
- To better address the needs of adolescents, who comprise the largest number of OVC, PEPFAR will increase efforts in youth livelihood development initiatives, focusing on higher levels of skill development. PEPFAR will also work to support

adolescents and young adults as they transition from OVC programs into society and careers.

PEPFAR is also working with countries to prioritize programming for most vulnerable children, including children living outside of family-based care; abused, exploited and neglected children; and children and adolescents who meet the criteria for other most-at-risk categories. Although these children account for only a small percentage of the total OVC population, they are often at higher risk for HIV infection, and less able to access traditional social service channels.

MOVING FORWARD WITH PROGRAMMING FOR ORPHANS AND VULNERABLE CHILDREN

Years 1-2

- Support countries to define, map, and plan a prioritized, multisectoral response to the needs of OVC populations and sub-populations within a country.
- Work with partner countries to identify gaps in capacity, including gaps in coordination among ministries overseeing education, food and nutrition, social welfare, and health.
- Establish training, mentoring, and technical assistance programs in partnership with governments in order to increase the number of professional staff in all agencies who can address cross-cutting OVC needs.
- Work with countries to increase support for family- based care by establishing and strengthening linkages between clinical and home- and community-based care.
- Scale up and ensure robust monitoring of existing high-impact OVC programs and support countries in developing, implementing, and evaluating innovative OVC pilot programming.
- Help countries ensure that policies for MARPs have adequate coverage and referrals for youth sub- populations.
- Support countries in developing a case management capability to assist the transition of young adults. from OVC services into society and careers.

Years 3-5

- Work with countries to engage in periodic and targeted surveys and other evaluations to determine impact of OVC programming.
- Ensure that countries have programs through which OVC can access livelihood development opportunities, including vocational training and microenterprise development training, to support themselves and their families.

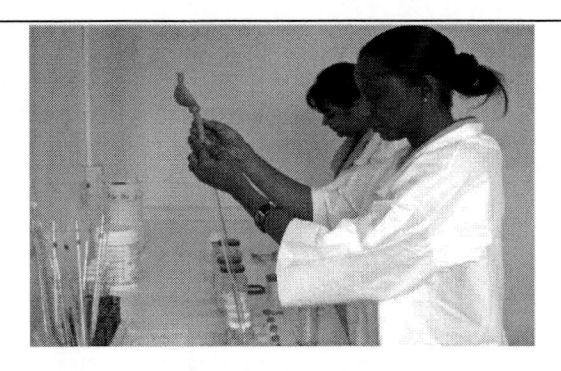

A risk for people needing medical care in many countries is the possibility of receiving sub-standard or counterfeit medicine. In March 2008, a PEPFAR-supported mini testing lab was established in Guyana to ensure drug quality. The laboratory is located in a warehouse setting and is managed by the resident pharmacist. Following training from the PEPFAR-supported Supply Chain Management System, staff now have the skills to test incoming pharmaceuticals to the Materials Management Unit, where all pharmaceuticals for the public sector are received and stored before being dispatched and distributed to health facilities. This unique arrangement of a quality testing post within a warehouse setting helps to assure the quality of all the pharmaceutical products distributed in the public health system.

TREATMENT

Key Points

- In partnership with country governments, PEPFAR is continuing scale-up of treatment, to directly support more than 4 million people in its next phase.
- PEPFAR is working with countries to reach a threshold of 85% ARV prophylaxis or treatment of those pregnant women found to be HIV-infected, in order to optimize maternal health and maximize HIV-free infant survival.
- In generalized epidemics, PEPFAR is working to reach a target of 65% early infection diagnosis, and support treatment for pediatric populations at a level commensurate with their representation in a larger country epidemic.
- Through country- and global-level efforts, PEPFAR is creating increased sustainability and capacity in treatment efforts and supporting countries in mobilizing and coordinating resources from multiple donors.
- PEPFAR is working with countries and international partners to expand identification and implementation of efficiencies in treatment, while ensuring continued expansion of measures to maintain adherence, quality, and retention in care.
- As part of the GHI, PEPFAR is integrating its treatment programs with prevention and care portfolios, other health programs, and larger development efforts.

Treatment has been the major success of PEPFAR. Prior to its creation in 2003, only about 50,000 individuals were on treatment in all sub-Saharan Africa. Six years later,

PEPFAR is supporting more than 2.4 million people on treatment worldwide. By combining the delivery of lifesaving drugs with strong adherence support, PEPFAR's drug compliance and efficacy rates are equivalent to those in the United States. A May 2009 study published in the *Annals of Internal Medicine* found that HIV-related mortality rates had dropped by 10.5% in the PEPFAR countries analyzed by researchers – implying that about 1.2 million deaths were averted due to PEPFAR.[8] Despite overwhelming odds, PEPFAR's first five years amply demonstrated that complicated treatment regimens can be delivered in a range of low-resource settings. The challenge of the next phase is to build the conditions through which to create eventual sustainability in PEPFAR's treatment programs.

Further increasing the global challenges in meeting treatment needs are data suggesting greater clinical benefits for individuals starting therapy earlier in the course of their infection. The WHO recently released a recommendation to initiate treatment at a CD4 cell count of $350/mm^3$, rather than $200/mm^3$. PEPFAR will continue to scale up its treatment programming in a manner that emphasizes health systems strengthening and creation of country- level capacity.

The benefits of treatment remain abundantly clear; people on treatment have improved immune function, resulting in fewer opportunistic diseases such as TB. People on treatment also have lower viral loads, which dramatically reduces transmissibility of the virus. There has been a significant decrease in hospital admissions due to wider availability of ARVs. Treatment extends lives, keeps families together, allows workers to continue and return to jobs, and reduces the number of OVCs. Research is also under way to determine the prevention impacts of treatment upon communities and populations. Finally, PEPFAR's programs have significant diplomatic benefits, increasing goodwill among the communities who have seen the impact of treatment.

Over its next phase, PEPFAR is configuring its treatment programs to achieve the following goals:

Targeting treatment

PEPFAR will continue to achieve major health impacts by expanding access to treatment, with a particular emphasis on the following:

Reaching the sickest first

Millions of people with CD4 cell counts under $200/mm^3$ are not currently reached by treatment. Within the context of national priorities, PEPFAR is making it a priority to reach the sickest individuals first, in order to prevent as many immediate deaths as possible. In countries with high coverage rates that are expanding eligibility, PEPFAR is helping to provide technical assistance and support for the overall treatment infrastructure. Given that many individuals are only tested once they become symptomatic, PEPFAR is also expanding country efforts to better link testing and counseling with treatment and care.

Pregnant women

In its next phase, PEPFAR will continue to intensify its focus on PMTCT as part of its prevention portfolio. In conjunction with that effort, PEPFAR supports countries in plans to expand treatment to pregnant women. Such a move not only prevents perinatal transmission, but also better sustains the health of the mother, resulting in additional positive impacts on her family's health and well-being.

PEPFAR is working to link and integrate broader antenatal care services with counseling, testing and treatment for pregnant women. Over its next phase, PEPFAR will work with countries to achieve 85% ARV prophylaxis or treatment of eligible pregnant women found to be HIV- infected. By targeting pregnant women, PEPFAR can also increase identification of and service provision to children HIV-positive mothers.

HIV/TB coinfected populations

TB is the leading cause of death for HIV-infected individuals, but identifying, treating, and preventing TB can dramatically reduce morbidity and mortality among those with HIV. PEPFAR is aggressively expanding its TB screening and HIV testing efforts to identify and treat coinfected individuals. PEPFAR is also working with countries to implement interventions to reduce the development of active TB and transmission of TB disease among those most at risk.

Supporting country-level coordination

In order to achieve the long-term goal of country-level sustainability, PEPFAR is increasing support to build country-level capacity to carry out national testing strategies. UNAIDS has been working with country partners to help define country-level need and develop estimates. It is now important to enable country-driven efforts to identify and to marshal multiple sources of funding to meet these treatment needs. PEPFAR is supporting technical assistance to countries as they work toward strategic adoption of new treatment guidelines, based on available programmatic capacity and country priorities. Over its next phase, PEPFAR will support country-level efforts to coordinate and integrate multiple sources of bilateral and multilateral treatment support. Doing so breaks down duplication and determines ways to jointly address the global need.

Increasing impact of pretreatment care and ensuring quality antiretroviral therapy programs

As part of efforts to work with countries to identify and implement effective and efficient practices, PEPFAR is assisting countries to aggressively prevent, identify, and treat opportunistic infections prior to the start of ARV treatment. With this activity, PLWHAs remain healthier longer, thus delaying the need for treatment. Once PEPFAR initiates treatment, programs work to maximize drug adherence and retention in care. Effective measures for doing so include use of pharmacy records and targeted monitoring, with a focus on gaining the greatest utility from first-line medications.

PEPFAR is working to detect acquired drug resistance and develop strategies to respond to this resistance. These efforts of PEPFAR will be closely linked to the efforts of other partners such as the Global Fund to Fight AIDS, Tuberculosis, and Malaria (Global Fund), UNAIDS, and the Gates Foundation to improve programmatic quality and better achieve "value for money." In its next phase, PEPFAR will also increase engagement of multilateral organizations, regional actors, private foundations and companies, and partner governments, among others, to address legal and regulatory barriers to the availability of high quality, inexpensive HIV-related commodities from local or international sources.

Expanding integration of treatment with both PEPFAR and other health programs

Treatment programs are not just clinical interventions, but opportunities to incorporate a holistic range of the health services needed to improve outcomes and quality of life for PLWHA. PEPFAR supports countries in efforts to coordinate and leverage treatment with prevention, care, and other health programs, as appropriate. In the next phase, PEPFAR treatment programs can serve as a platform to link to health services, including:

Integration with PEPFAR prevention and care services

PEPFAR treatment programs are often already integrated with pre-antiretroviral treatment (ART) services for PLWHA. Many PEPFAR treatment programs are used as a point to engage in Health, Dignity, and Prevention Programs for PLWHA, their partners, and their families. PEPFAR is working with countries to integrate treatment with standard packages of pre-ART, essential support services, and necessary prevention services for PLWHAs and their families.

Integration with other health and development programs

In many of the countries where PEPFAR works, clients and their families also suffer from malnutrition, TB, malaria, and other chronic progressive conditions requiring medical attention. HIV-positive women need routine reproductive health services. Their children need preventive care, like immunizations, and diagnosis and treatment of illnesses, like diarrhea and pneumonia. PEPFAR treatment programs will be used as a platform from which to build linkages to multiple primary and specialty health services. Doing so increases community-level access to quality care and reduces the stigma associated with HIV. Care and treatment will serve as one component of a clinic's broader service capacity, and clinics can be used as the base for referrals to community-based supportive services for PLWHA and their families.

Addressing the needs of vulnerable populations

There are specific populations that require additional considerations when transitioning them into treatment, including the following:

Pediatric populations

It is estimated that by two years of age, over 50% of children infected with HIV will have died in the absence of treatment.[9] New pediatric HIV infections have become exceedingly rare in the U.S. due to the rapid expansion of effective ARV prophylaxis and treatment to HIV-infected pregnant women. PEPFAR supports making such infections equally rare in the developing world. However, the millions of children already living with HIV or newly infected with HIV need a range of services to stay alive and thrive.

PEPFAR is working to support treatment for pediatric populations at a level commensurate with their representation in a larger country epidemic. For example, based on prevalence surveys, if children represent 10% of the PLWHA population in a given country, PEPFAR should also strive to ensure that they represent 10% of those on ARV treatment in that country.

In order to provide treatment to infants, PEPFAR and other funders must continue to scale up early infant diagnosis and laboratory referral networks that produce rapid results for use by clinicians. PEPFAR is focusing on reaching a target of 65% early infant diagnosis, enabling newly diagnosed infants to receive care and treatment. PEPFAR is also working with countries to ensure that 80% of older children of HIV-positive mothers are tested and referred to care and treatment as necessary.

Marginalized populations

The stigma, discrimination, and marginalization faced by most-at-risk populations often extends into the health care system. In its next phase, PEPFAR will renew efforts to ensure its supported treatment programs are responsive to the needs of marginalized populations. PEPFAR is working with countries to expand linkages between prevention, treatment and care programs that address the needs of these populations. Examples include opioid substitution therapy as necessary for HIV-positive IDUs, or post-exposure prophylaxis for those who have experienced sexual assault. PEPFAR will also supporting efforts to ensure that health care workers are trained to protect patient confidentiality and provide nonjudgmental services. Finally, given that these groups are often ones that do not receive attention at a national level, PEPFAR is working with governments to incorporate their needs into national treatment plans.

MOVING FORWARD WITH TREATMENT

Years 1-2

- Work with countries to determine need and identify plans for addressing country-level treatment burden among multiple donors, and support their efforts to engage in oversight and management of treatment programs.
- Scale-up treatment with an emphasis on reaching key populations.
- Support efforts to increase aggressive treatment of opportunistic infections, and maximize the impact of first-line ART through effective adherence and retention measures.
- Support country efforts to identify and expand access to lower-cost drugs.
- Expand effective referral systems and linkages between HIV prevention, care, and treatment services, as well as broader health and development services.

Years 3 -5

- Assist countries with high levels of coverage to transition to increased ownership of programming.
- Continue support for country, regional, and multilateral efforts to identify and expand access to lower-cost drugs.
- Implement efficiencies resulting from increased integration.

ACRONYMS AND ABBREVIATIONS

ART   Antiretroviral Treatment
ARV   Antiretroviral Drug
BCC   Behavior Change Communication **CSI** Child Status Index
FP   Family Planning
GHI   Global Health Initiative
Global Fund   Global Fund to Fight AIDS, Tuberculosis, and Malaria
IDU   Injecting Drug User
IEC   Information, Education and Communication
KAIS   Kenya AIDS Indicator Survey
MAT   Medication-Assisted Therapy
MC   Male Circumcision
MCP   Multiple and Concurrent Sexual Partnerships
MDR-TB   Multi-Drug-Resistant Tuberculosis
MARPs   Most-at-Risk Populations
MSM   Men Who Have Sex with Men
OVC   Orphans and Vulnerable Children
PEP   Post-Exposure Prophylaxis
PEPFAR   U.S. President's Emergency Plan for AIDS Relief
PLWHA   People Living with HIV/AIDS
PMTCT   Prevention of Mother-to-Child HIV transmission
UNAIDS   Joint United Nations Programme on HIV/AIDS
UNODC   United Nations Office on Drugs and Crime
USG   United States Government
WFP   World Food Program
WHO   World Health Organization
XDR-TB   Extensively Drug-Resistant Tuberculosis

End Notes

[1] http://data.unaids.org/pub/PressRelease/2009/20091124_PR_EpiUpdate_en.pdf
[2] http://www.unaids.org/en/CountryResponses/UniversalAccess/default.asp
[3] http://www.who.int/hiv/topics/malecircumcision/en/index.html
[4] http://data.unaids.org/pub/GlobalReport/2008/jc1510_2008_global_report_pp29_62_en.pdf
[5] http://www.unodc.org/documents/hiv-aids/WHO   %20Target%20Setting%20Guide%20-%20FINAL%20-%20Feb%2009.pdf
[6] http://www.unicef.org/publications/files/cob_layout6-013.pdf, p 7, 3
[7] http://siteresources.worldbank.org/INTHIVAIDS/Resources/375798-1103037153392/ReachingOuttoAfricasOrphans.pdf, p 36
[8] http://www.annals.org/cgi/content/full/0000605-200905190-00117v1
[9] Newell ML, Coovadia H, Cortina-Borja M, Rollins N, Gaillard P, Dabis F. Mortality of infected and uninfected infants born to HIV-infected mothers in Africa: a pooled analysis. Lancet 2004; 364: 1236 – 1243.

In: Global HIV/AIDS Threat and the U.S. Response
Editor: David R. Carmody

ISBN: 978-1-61324-568-2
© 2011 Nova Science Publishers, Inc.

Chapter 4

THE U.S. PRESIDENT'S EMERGENCY PLAN FOR AIDS RELIEF (FIVE-YEAR STRATEGY): ANNEX-PEPFAR AND THE GLOBAL CONTEXT OF HIV

David R. Carmody

PARTNERSHIP FRAMEWORKS

In July 2008, as part of its reauthorization, the U.S. President's Emergency Plan for AIDS Relief (PEPFAR) was encouraged to negotiate framework documents with partner countries. By establishing these partnerships, PEPFAR is promoting and developing a more sustainable approach to the fight against HIV/AIDS at the country level. These Partnership Frameworks are characterized by strengthened country capacity, ownership, and leadership, and represent a substantially new focus for PEPFAR. Partnership Frameworks pave the way for approaches to foreign assistance based upon collaboration on principles that are common to U.S. Government (USG) objectives and partner country plans and activities.

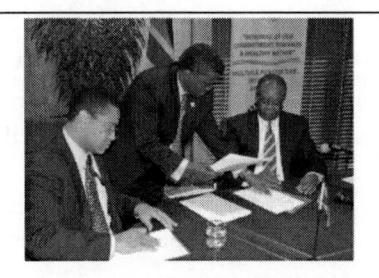

On June 4, 2009, Maurice S. Parker, U.S. Ambassador to Swaziland, and Dr. Barnabas S. Dlamini, Prime Minister of the Kingdom of Swaziland, signed the Swaziland Partnership Framework on HIV and AIDS for 2009-2013. The Partnership Framework focuses on the development of a comprehensive national HIV prevention program, improving the coverage and quality of HIV-related treatment and care, mitigating the impacts of HIV/AIDS with a focus on children, increasing access to high quality medical male circumcision, and building the human and institutional capacity needed to achieve and sustain these goals.

Partnership Frameworks provide a joint five-year strategy for cooperation between the USG and the partner government, with the participation of other partners. In some instances, PEPFAR is also negotiating Partnership Frameworks at the regional level. Each Framework clearly establishes plans for provision of technical assistance and support for service delivery, policy development, and coordinated financial commitments. At the end of the five-year timeframe, in addition to gains around HIV prevention, care, and treatment, country governments will be better positioned to assume responsibility for their national responses to the epidemic.

Like other aspects of PEPFAR, the development of Partnership Frameworks is an interagency effort. It is carried out under the authority of the U.S. Global AIDS Coordinator at the Department of State, and led by the U.S. Ambassador in-country with support from the interagency PEPFAR country team. The process of negotiating these partnerships also involves the active participation of other key partners from civil society.

The primary lessons learned to date include the following, which PEPFAR will use to guide the process moving forward:

- It is critical to involve high-level, broad representation from multiple ministries in the partner government from the very beginning;
- Where applicable, Partnership Frameworks should build upon existing national strategies;
- While the central dialogue in a Framework is between the USG and the partner government, multisectoral involvement ensures buy-in from all involved parties across government and civil society, including people living with HIV/AIDS (PLWHA);
- Continuous, ongoing dialogue allows all voices to be heard and issues to be rapidly resolved as they arise; and
- The process of negotiating these documents provides a new and welcome platform for leveraging policy reforms.

The principles used to guide the development of these partnerships include the following:

- **Country ownership:** Governments must be at the center of decision-making, leadership, and management of their national HIV/AIDS programs and health systems. Over the period defined in the Partnership Framework, as appropriate in the respective country, PEPFAR-supported programs will take steps to progressively shift supported activities from direct implementation to technical assistance. These efforts will build government and local capacity to plan, oversee, and manage programs, deliver services, and coordinate assistance from multiple donors. Discussions regarding country ownership should involve Ministries of Health and all appropriate ministries and high level elected officials that impact HIV/AIDS programming. As noted above, local civil society is also a key component in multisectoral discussions. By including the contributions of multiple donors as part of the Framework, PEPFAR will help countries take a position of leadership in coordinating among funders.

- **Sustainability:** Partnership Frameworks should be crafted to help ensure that the national response to the HIV/AIDS epidemic is moving toward sustainability while improving quality of programming. Efforts to create sustainability must support the country government in developing the capacity to manage all relevant components of a multisector health system. Donor funding should supplement, not supplant, existing country work around HIV/AIDS, and Frameworks should account for the contributions of public, private, and civil society organizations.
- **Flexibility:** Different approaches to Partnership Frameworks are appropriate for different settings. Country context must drive Framework objectives and approaches. Thus, the appropriate mix of direct services, health systems strengthening, and technical assistance will vary by country within the context of national strategies and plans. In addition, the policy areas addressed by Partnership Frameworks should reflect the specific policy development needs of the relevant country.
- **Progress toward policy reform and increased management and financial accountability:** Partnership Frameworks emphasize key policies that promote effective, sustainable, and quality HIV/AIDS programs. They also offer an important new opportunity to engage government partners in commitments. Through these Frameworks, PEPFAR and government partners emphasize overall accountability for resources and appropriate budgeting in HIV/AIDS programs.
- **Integration of HIV/AIDS into strengthened health systems and a broader health and development agenda:** Partnership Frameworks contribute to strengthened HIV/AIDS services within the context of the broader health system. In an environment with diverse development needs, they promote integration of services to maximize impact and efficiency.
- **Monitoring and evaluation (M&E):** Partnership Frameworks set measurable goals, objectives, and concrete commitments for PEPFAR, the government, and all partners in the Partnership Framework. The Partnership Framework identifies indicators to assess progress toward achieving these goals and objectives, and meeting national commitments.
- **"Do no harm":** Partnership Frameworks promote sustainability and country ownership through capacity-building of governments and local partners. Existing service systems supported by PEPFAR and partner governments are continuing to deliver quality prevention, treatment, and care services while the transition to country ownership occurs over time.

IMPROVING RESOURCE MANAGEMENT AND MOBILIZATION

Key Points

- It is necessary to mount a true global response to the shared global burden of unmet need.
- PEPFAR is identifying efficiencies and opportunities for leveraging in programming; the cost-savings gained from these efficiencies can expand the reach of the program.

- Funding will be targeted to build upon successes and established systems and achieve greater impact.
- PEPFAR remains committed to working with countries in addressing both generalized and concentrated epidemics.
- An immediate priority of PEPFAR is to support country-level, regional, and global efforts to review prevention, care and treatment needs, as well as ways to jointly marshal resources to meet the global need.
- PEPFAR is building the capacity of country governments to serve as the conveners and coordinators of diverse funding sources.

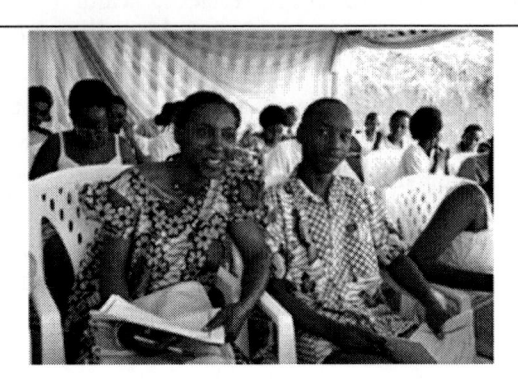

In Rwanda, 67 percent of the population is under the age of 20 and approximately two in five people report becoming sexually active before age 20. While nearly all young adults in Rwanda are aware of HIV/AIDS, less than 50 percent of 15- to 19-year-olds have an in-depth understanding of the disease. To address this concern, a PEPFAR-supported program began training secondary students and their parents on how to talk openly about HIV/AIDS and other health issues. Through this program, families participate in five sessions that are designed to break down communication barriers and encourage safe behavior. Upon completion of the training, these students and parents become role models in their communities, passing on the information and methods they have learned to their peers.

From 2004 to 2009, the USG has contributed an unprecedented amount to global HIV/AIDS programs. Despite the significant gains in health outcomes that have resulted from these investments, there is still unmet need that outstrips the ability of any single donor to meet it.

According to the World Health Organization (WHO), while more than 4 million people are receiving antiretroviral therapy in low- and middle-income countries, more than 5 million people in these countries are currently in need of treatment.[1] The WHO recently released clinical guidelines that recommend treatment initiation at a CD4 cell count of $350/mm^3$, rather than $200/mm^3$. These guidelines are expected to roughly double the number of people in need of treatment. In addition, the impact of treatment on transmission and future incidence is currently under active debate at the WHO and the Joint United Nations Programme on HIV/AIDS (UNAIDS).

UNAIDS has done significant work in establishing estimates for long-term funding needs. These estimates inform efforts to meet the Millennium Development Goal of halting and reversing the spread of HIV by 2015. According to UNAIDS, the needs for 2010, based upon country-defined targets in low- and middle-income countries, will be $25.1 billion. This figure encompasses at least $11.6 billion needed for prevention, $7 billion needed for treatment and care, and $2.5 billion for programs serving orphans and vulnerable children.[2] In 2008, according to UNAIDS, $13.7 billion was available for HIV programming in low- and middle-income countries.[3] Given the scope and enormity of need, a coordinated global effort is necessary to mount an effective and sustainable response to the epidemic. To contribute to this type of response, PEPFAR is focusing on the following:

- Identifying efficiencies;
- Targeting funding to build upon successes and achieve greater impact; and
- Supporting countries in identifying and marshaling additional resources for their HIV epidemic.

Efficiencies in Programming and Systems

Efforts to combat global HIV/AIDS have benefited from significant funding over the past decade, allowing for the establishment and rapid scale-up of services. As PEPFAR transitions to a sustainable response, it is working to identify and implement efficiencies at both field and headquarters levels. Since PEPFAR was created, investments from the USG, partner countries, and governments have created conditions that reduce the overall costs associated with programming, particularly the provision of antiretroviral drugs (ARVs). These conditions include:

Investing in equipment, infrastructure, training

Overall, per-patient financial costs of treatment have dropped as global AIDS efforts have matured. Much of the infrastructure and equipment required for a site to function was established before patients were enrolled, and any expansion in patient numbers was preceded by expansions in clinic capacity. As PEPFAR works with the Global Health Initiative (GHI) to expand and build health systems, it will build upon the country infrastructure platform to continue to reduce costs for increased coverage of care.

Improving personnel response

PEPFAR programs benefited from economies of scale as patient cohorts expanded. Increasing numbers of patients are often treated by the same number of health workers as a result of several factors, such as improved worker efficiency after the start-up period. More recently, there is some early indication of the effects of task-shifting upon improving efficiencies. Over the next phase, PEPFAR is identifying additional efficiencies to assist health workers to care for patients. Through the GHI, it will also explore mechanisms like appropriate co-location of services to reduce recurring personnel and facility costs.

Decreasing commodity costs

Licensing, approval, and competitive manufacture of generic formulations of ARVs has resulted in an environment of rapidly declining pricing for these commodities. PEPFAR, utilizing bulk-purchasing mechanisms, has been aggressive in taking advantage of these lower

ARV prices to extend treatment to additional patients. PEPFAR is working with partner countries and existing multilateral and foundation efforts to encourage the policy changes needed to continue this downward trajectory of drug prices. As part of the GHI, PEPFAR will also explore possible efficiencies in supply chain management.

Marshaling Resources for Need

The USG is the major funder of global HIV/AIDS programming. As of 2007, it contributed at least 51% of international donor government assistance to HIV/AIDS.[4] The majority of this funding is directed through PEPFAR's bilateral programs. USG contributions also account for roughly 29% of Global Fund resources directed to AIDS.[5] Because of the scope of the epidemic, an effective response to global AIDS requires funding from multiple sources, including country governments, bilateral donors, regional actors, multilateral partners, private foundations, and nongovernmental organizations. To support a diverse funding base, PEPFAR is building the capacity of country governments to serve as the conveners and coordinators of these diverse funding sources.

An immediate priority of PEPFAR is to support countries in reassessing and identifying the scale of their national HIV/AIDS epidemic, to ensure interventions respond to existing and emerging realities. Governments should convene or expand inclusive processes in which demographic data is used to define and prioritize unmet need. Once the government has defined need and set priorities for action, PEPFAR will support the country in efforts to coordinate donors and investments. PEPFAR is encouraging its multilateral partners, including the Global Fund and UNAIDS, to join similar coordinated assessments and processes at the national and international level.

Through the GHI, PEPFAR will explore possible financing and leveraging opportunities beyond those traditionally utilized in USG development assistance, including those involving public-private partnerships. PEPFAR will also expand its cooperation with multilateral partners to explore possible cooperation around internationally-supported financing mechanisms.

Country and Regional Overview

When PEPFAR was created, investments were focused in 15 focus countries, although program funding was utilized to support efforts to combat HIV/AIDS in areas beyond these 15 countries. In the next phase of PEPFAR, the program will work to reduce the distinction between "focus" and "other" countries. While the former focus countries account for a significant amount of program funding, PEPFAR has made significant investments in over 30 countries and regions. These countries include both those where the epidemic is concentrated among specific populations, and those where HIV occurs among the general population. In many countries where HIV prevalence rates are above 1% - the widely defined threshold for generalized epidemics – prevalence is often much higher among sub-populations, such as men who have sex with men (MSM) and sex workers. PEPFAR's regional approaches provide an ability to review and apply best practices among similar countries. Whether the countries and regions where PEPFAR works have generalized or concentrated epidemics, all these places have unmet need in HIV prevention, care, and treatment.

Given the dynamic nature of the epidemic, PEPFAR will ensure that its programs are flexible and tailored to the country context. This context includes not only epidemiologic data, but the need to coordinate and reduce duplication with multilateral and country partners and build upon existing health systems. It is important to note that PEPFAR's response is likely to vary based upon the level of investments that exist from PEPFAR and other donor sources within a country. For example, in a country with a concentrated epidemic, PEPFAR's work may focus on providing technical assistance to governments and working to coordinate with mechanisms of the Global Fund to Fight AIDS, Tuberculosis, and Malaria (Global Fund). Alternately, in a low-resource hyperendemic country, PEPFAR's work may focus on ensuring quality service delivery and strengthening country capacity to deliver care.

A brief summary of the epidemic profile in the countries and regions where PEPFAR works follows. Country-level prevalence estimates are from the 2008 UNAIDS Report on the global AIDS epidemic:[6]

Africa

Southern Africa, the epicenter of the pandemic, has countries with the highest HIV prevalence rates in the world, including Swaziland (26%), Botswana (24%), and Lesotho (23%). In these "hyperendemic" countries, HIV has spread widely across the population. The region also has the largest number of PLWHA. Infection rates vary substantially within countries, and there are significant gender disparities in prevalence in the 15-24 age cohort.

HIV infection rates appear to be stabilizing in many countries in Southern Africa, but are still at high levels.[7] Declines and plateaus likely reflect the natural course of the epidemic as well as the contribution of program interventions. The potential impact of treatment roll-out on prevention also remains unclear. More analysis is needed to better understand the factors contributing to evolving epidemic trends.

In **West Africa,** HIV prevalence is notably lower than in southern Africa. High-prevalence West African countries include Côte d'Ivoire (4%) and Nigeria (3%). This lower regional prevalence is likely attributable to numerous factors, especially much higher prevalence of male circumcision.

HIV prevalence in **East Africa** falls between the levels in West and Southern Africa. Trends in prevalence vary, but there is evidence that prevalence has stabilized.[8] Urban prevalence tends to be higher than rural, but access to services is still needed in rural areas.

Caribbean and Latin America

In the **Caribbean**, many low-level generalized epidemics have stabilized, with evidence of slight declines among some sub-populations. However, prevalence rates remain high in certain countries, including Haiti (2.2%). In **Latin America**, most countries are experiencing concentrated epidemics, although some countries like Guyana (2.5%) have higher prevalence rates. In these areas, the main mode of HIV transmission is heterosexual sex, often tied to transactional sex, although emerging evidence indicates that substantial transmission is also occurring among men who have sex with men.[9]

Southeast and East Asia

PEPFAR is operating in several countries throughout **Southeast and East Asia**. Thailand has the highest prevalence rate in Asia (1.4%). However, the large populations of many countries within Asia mean that a low prevalence rate may translate into a large number of people living with the virus. Approximately 4.7 million people in this region are living with HIV, the second highest number outside of sub-Saharan Africa.[10] PEPFAR will continue to support treatment in low-income countries in this region, while also working with governments and civil society to address barriers to services among marginalized populations. In emerging economies like India, where prevalence rates are still low but the number of people living with HIV is substantial, PEPFAR will expand technical assistance and work to leverage investments of multilateral mechanisms like the Global Fund.

Eastern Europe and Central Asia

In **Eastern Europe and Central Asia,** there is a significant need to address concentrated epidemics, with high rates of HIV occurring among injecting drug users and sex workers. Countries in this area with higher prevalence rates include Ukraine (1.6%) and the Russian Federation (1.1%). PEPFAR will continue to work with countries to support technical assistance and policy reform to address the needs of these often-marginalized populations. PEPFAR will also work to leverage existing investments of these countries and multilateral mechanisms like the Global Fund.

MOVING FORWARD WITH IMPROVING RESOURCE MANAGEMENT AND MOBILIZATION

Years 1-2

- Identify and implement efficiencies at field and headquarters levels, including those that lower the cost of treatment.
- Support countries to reassess and identify the scale of their national HIV/AIDS epidemic to ensure interventions respond to existing and emerging realities.
- Build the capacity of country governments to serve as the conveners and coordinators of diverse funding sources, and encourage multilateral efforts to coordinate donors and investments at the international level.
- Through the GHI, explore possible financing and leveraging opportunities beyond those traditionally utilized in USG development assistance, including those involving public-private partnerships.
- Identify ways in which existing health systems and infrastructure can be utilized in efforts to reduce costs and increase access.

Years 3-5

- Use existing and emerging data to ensure continued and coordinated alignment of PEPFAR investments with country-identified needs and plans.

- Transition resources from direct service provision to financing of and technical assistance for country- managed mechanisms, where feasible.

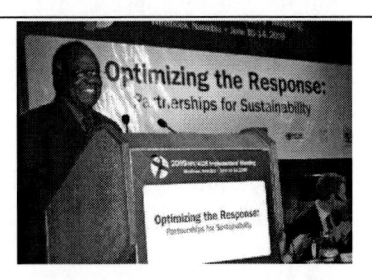

H.E Hifikepunye Pohamba, President of the Republic of Namibia, opened the 2009 HIV/AIDS Implementers' Meeting in Windhoek, Namibia on June 10, 2009. The meeting was hosted by the Government of Namibia and co-sponsored by PEPFAR; the Global Fund to Fight AIDS, Tuberculosis and Malaria; UNAIDS; UNICEF; the World Bank; the World Health Organization; and the Global Network of People Living with HIV. The conference focused on three major themes: sustainability, efficiency and effectiveness, and prevention.

STRENGTHENING AND LEVERAGING KEY MULTILATERAL INSTITUTIONS

Key Points

- PEPFAR's success is linked to the success of its multilateral partners, particularly the Global Fund.
- Through the GHI, the USG will expand engagement with key multilateral institutions and global health partnerships in support of a comprehensive approach to achieving the Millennium Development Goals (MDG) and other core objectives.
- In order to ensure the long-term sustainability of the Global Fund, PEPFAR will support reforms that create conditions for eventual transition of some PEPFAR programs to Global Fund mechanisms.
- PEPFAR will support efforts by UNAIDS to mobilize global action and facilitate adoption of country-level changes that allow for rapid scale-up of key interventions.
- Given the important role of WHO as the key normative global health institution, PEPFAR is working to expand collaboration and promote best practices with this organization.
- PEPFAR will expand efforts to coordinate with multilateral development banks and support their health systems investments.

Since the inception of PEPFAR, the USG has considered both bilateral and multilateral efforts essential in achieving durable success in the fight against AIDS. PEPFAR needs to work with and through others to build political will, establish international norms, ensure a broad-based multisectoral response, and support service delivery. In addition, through its work with multilateral partners, PEPFAR is able to leverage its investments, mobilize resources, and provide stable external financing.

The need for a coordinated multilateral response is even greater today than it was five years ago. As PEPFAR shifts from an emergency response, it is expanding work with multilateral organizations and bilateral partners, and increasing country-level and international commitment to financing and implementation.

The Obama administration is committed to a collaborative, transparent, and integrated approach to international health and development challenges. PEPFAR's success is linked to the success of multilateral mechanisms like the Global Fund and multilateral partners like the UN system.

Over the next phase of PEPFAR, the program is working toward an international consensus on the scale of the global HIV/AIDS need, as well as the increased political and financial commitments necessary to meet it.

Global Fund to Fight AIDS, Tuberculosis, and Malaria

The Global Fund is a unique global public-private partnership dedicated to attracting and disbursing resources to prevent and treat AIDS, tuberculosis, and malaria. As a partnership among governments, civil society, the private sector and affected communities, the Global Fund represents a new approach to international health financing.

Since its creation in 2002 and with strong financial support from the USG, the Global Fund has become the main external financing mechanism for programs to fight AIDS, tuberculosis, and malaria. It has approved funding of $18.7 billion for more than 600 grant programs in 144 countries. Worldwide, of all international financing, the Global Fund provides approximately one quarter for AIDS, two-thirds for tuberculosis, and three quarters for malaria.

PEPFAR strongly supports the Global Fund. The United States made the founding contribution to the Global Fund, and remains its largest donor. The USG has contributed more than $4.3 billion to the Global Fund to date, with additional pledges that bring the total USG commitment through fiscal year 2009 to $4.5 billion. In addition to these direct contributions, PEPFAR provides specific technical assistance funding for grant implementation and oversight. By working through the Global Fund, the USG can catalyze contributions from other donors, expand the geographic reach of USG bilateral programs, promote country ownership, and increase the sustainability of national health programs.

The Global Fund model represents an inherently country-owned approach, which fits well with PEPFAR's goal of supporting increased country ownership of national HIV/AIDS programs. This goal is critical to the long-term sustainability of AIDS responses and can be supported through a robust and coordinated multilateral response. PEPFAR is working with both the Global Fund and the UN system to support increased country ownership in a coordinated manner. The Global Fund can provide countries with predictable, performance-based financing, and the UN system has the mandate, country presence, and expertise to build country-level capacity and leadership. Nevertheless, continued USG engagement and support at the country level will be essential in supporting a full transition to country ownership. Consequently, PEPFAR will expand the engagement of its country teams with its country-level Global Fund counterparts and processes.

PEPFAR is also supporting a shift in Global Fund grant architecture. This shift would move it from a project- based approach to a program-based approach supporting comprehensive national responses to AIDS, tuberculosis, and malaria. These reforms are intended to consolidate and rationalize country programs and reporting requirements, harmonize Global Fund financing with country- level fiscal and planning cycles, and reduce transaction costs. By reducing duplication of effort at the country level, both PEPFAR and the Global Fund will enable countries to identify gaps in services, and achieve better value for money.

PEPFAR's long-term goal is to see more management and operation of bilateral programs conducted by the countries themselves, with financial support through the Global Fund. In order to promote this goal, PEPFAR is working to improve grant performance, quality, and consistency of services, and transparent and accountable financial management. PEPFAR is continuing efforts with the Global Fund Secretariat, its Inspector General, and its Board to improve the impact, oversight, and cost-effectiveness of Global Fund grants. Financial and program accountability is paramount to ensuring that PEPFAR funds are effectively leveraged and that, ultimately, programs are successfully implemented.

Joint United Nations Programme on HIV/AIDS

UNAIDS is an innovative venture of the United Nations family, comprising a Geneva-based Secretariat and 10 cosponsoring bodies: the World Health Organization, the UN Development Programme, the UN Office on Drugs and Crime, the UN Children's Fund, the UN Population Fund, the International Labor Organization, the World Food Program, the UN High Commissioner for Refugees, the World Bank, and the UN Educational, Scientific, and Cultural Organization.

UNAIDS is guided by a Programme Coordinating Board (PCB) with representatives from 22 governments from all geographic regions, the UNAIDS Cosponsors, and ten representatives of nongovernmental organizations, including associations of people living with HIV. UNAIDS is widely viewed as UN reform in action.

UNAIDS has field-based staff and works directly in 70 countries, addressing HIV/AIDS primarily through country-coordination theme groups that seek to mobilize all sectors to address AIDS. The UN system is an important partner because of its power to convene. UNAIDS also provides technical support for country-led strategies, provides robust global-level strategic information, and ensures the meaningful involvement of civil society in efforts to combat the epidemic.

The gains made to date in the fight against AIDS are largely due to a multisectoral approach that recognizes both the clinical needs and structural contributors to the epidemic. The UN system is an essential part of this multisectoral and rights-based approach, and UNAIDS has been an effective mechanism within that system to mobilize and coordinate Member States. Increasingly, UNAIDS is at the forefront of global efforts to mobilize additional resources and forge coalitions to leverage the AIDS response in achieving broad-based health and development objectives.

In this next phase of PEPFAR, the USG will, as a board member and major funder of UNAIDS, continue to be a strong supporter of the organization. UNAIDS serves as the mechanism through which to organize and maintain momentum in the UN system's response to the epidemic. PEPFAR will partner with UNAIDS as a convener and norm-setter to facilitate increased action and attention in certain areas of the epidemic. In particular, PEPFAR views the UN system as able to contribute effectively to rapid scale-up of cross-cutting gender interventions, PMTCT, male circumcision, and prevention among injecting drug users (IDUs).

While most parts of the Joint Programme are not programmatic implementers, UNAIDS can establish and disseminate international norms, build political will, and provide technical support at the country level around these interventions. PEPFAR will also collaborate with UNAIDS to strengthen national ownership of the response to HIV and support a multilateral process to build upon country-level processes through which global need and global resources for the fight against HIV are identified.

World Health Organization

As the global norm-setting body for public health, WHO builds support for best practices, including PMTCT, and disseminating promising new interventions like male circumcision. The WHO provides technical support to governments, helping them develop National Strategies that include guidelines for minimum packages of services. In addition, the WHO is a global leader in the area of health systems strengthening. PEPFAR and WHO are discussing a four-year strategic framework that emphasizes, among other areas, collaboration in health systems strengthening, strategic information, antiretroviral treatment, prevention, and the challenges posed by HIV/TB coinfection. PEPFAR and WHO are continuing collaboration to promote best practices and make progress on a number of specific challenges related to the epidemic.

Multilateral Development Banks

Multilateral development banks like the World Bank and the International Monetary Fund play important roles in financing and economic and policy analysis that inform both HIV/AIDS work and broader development policy. In its next phase, PEPFAR will expand efforts to coordinatewith these organizations to improve the performanceof their health systems investments. It will also work tobetter integrate PEPFAR services with their broader economic development efforts.

MOVING FORWARD WITH STRENGTHENING AND LEVERAGING KEY MULTILATERAL INSTITUTIONS

Years 1-2

- Expand work with multilateral organizations and bilateral partners, increasing country-level and international commitment to financing and implementation.
- Support Global Fund efforts to shift grant architecture to program-based approach.

- Expand engagement with UNAIDS around gender, male circumcision, PMTCT, and comprehensive packages of care for IDUs.
- Complete development of PEPFAR/WHO strategic framework.
- Engage with multilateral development banks around health system investments.

Years 3-5

- Increase alignment of PEPFAR and Global Fund funding with national plans based upon new grant architecture.
- Harmonize PEPFAR, UNAIDS, and Global Fund indicators in support of country-level objectives.
- Continue efforts with multilateral partners in building country capacity to deliver services and manage distribution programs.

PUBLIC-PRIVATE PARTNERSHIPS

Secretary Clinton has said, "The problems we face today will not be solved by governments alone. It will be in partnerships – partnerships with philanthropy, with global business, partnerships with civil society." As PEPFAR shifts to promotion of country-led sustainable responses, it is essential to employ all possible mechanisms to build systems and expand capacity.

Public-Private Partnerships

Public-private partnerships (PPPs) are a tool that can enhance PEPFAR and country government approaches to HIV/AIDS and strengthening of overall health systems. PEPFAR has worked with public-private engagement mechanisms throughout the government, including the Department of State's Global Partnerships Initiative. Over the past three years, PEPFAR has made significant strides in brokering PPPs and establishing relationships with key private sector entities.

Private sector partners have skills that complement PEPFAR's technical focus, including marketing and distribution networks. Many of PEPFAR's private sector partners have specific technical expertise in areas such as laboratory capacity and information technology. PEPFAR has worked to link their capabilities with areas of program emphasis to leverage not just dollars, but results that can be sustained in the long term.

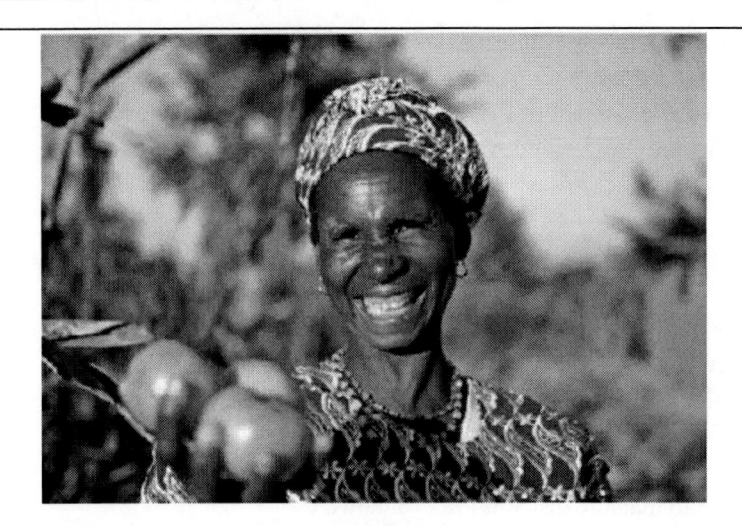

In September 2009, General Mills, a leading U.S. food company, PEPFAR and USAID launched a public-private partnership that will improve the capacity of small and medium-sized food businesses across sub-Saharan Africa to produce healthy, fortified food products and widen the availability of fortified flour products for people living with HIV enrolled in PEPFAR-supported "Food by Prescription" programs. Over time, the partnership aims to improve the ability of these small and medium-sized enterprises to produce quality, nutritious and safe food at affordable prices.

Over the next phase of PEPFAR, the program is developing partnerships that will deliver impact with low transac¬tion costs. There will be an emphasis on partnerships supporting prevention, broad health systems strengthening, and human resources for health. PEPFAR's PPP projects will explicitly integrate gender strategies as a cross-cut¬ting element wherever feasible. The following are ways that PPPs can support the vision for the next phase of PEPFAR:

- **Identifying and promoting integration of the private sector in service delivery.** According to a 2007 study conducted for the World Bank/IFC by McKinsey, around 60% of sub-Saharan Africa's total health expenditures were financed by private parties; about 65% of that was directed to for-profit providers.[11] This spending is not based on wealth. According to a compilation of Demographic and Health Surveys (DHS) from 10 sub-Saharan African countries, 44% of those in the poorest quintile brought their sick children to private, for-profit, providers.[12] PEPFAR must work with partner governments to help them identify and understand the role that private and non-profit providers currently play in the response to the disease. Doing so allows governments to coordinate with these private partners as part of a comprehensive national health system.
- **Facilitating provision of technical assistance in areas of core competencies.** The private sector can work directly with government officials and healthcare workers to build their capacity and strengthen national health systems. As PEPFAR focuses on increasing capacity-building and technical assistance to governments, it can help to

facilitate relationships between partner countries and businesses supporting development of core competencies.

- **Supporting North-South and South-South mentoring programs.** Part of PEPFAR's PPP mandate is to engage professional organizations and companies, diaspora groups, and even individuals involved in PEPFAR programs. Leading HIV/AIDS experts, clinicians, nurses, and practitioners in the United States can play an important collaborative role with their counterparts in PEPFAR countries. Over the next phase of PEPFAR, the program is expanding collaborative and mentoring relationships with partner governments.

- **Expanding and integrating workplace programs.** In many countries, businesses were and are on the leading edge of the response to HIV/AIDS, given the threat that the epidemic poses to the stability of the local economy. However, the development of workplace programs has not always been linked to a national HIV/ AIDS prevention response. Private companies can play a leading role in the sustained response to the disease through the workplace, but a new, up-to-date strategy for engagement needs to be developed. PEPFAR can help governments ascertain the landscape of workplace programs and attain efficiencies by ensuring coordination of workplace efforts with larger public programming.

- **Integrating gender strategies.** PPPs play an important role in PEPFAR's gender programming strategy. PEPFAR engages with private companies to address structural issues that impact women and men's risk for HIV infection and access to quality care and treatment. The private sector can play a strong role in mobilizing investment capital to support women's access to income and productive resources. With increased emphasis from both PEPFAR and external actors on gender-based violence, PEPFAR is working to develop partnerships around this specific issue. PEPFAR can also do more to engage women as both providers and recipients of private sector health services. These private services must be strategically linked to reproductive health, family planning, and maternal care, and serve as a conduit to get families into HIV and other health services.

ACRONYMS AND ABBREVIATIONS

ART	Antiretroviral Treatment
ARV	Antiretroviral Drug
DHS	Demographic and Health Survey
GHI	Global Health Initiative
Global Fund	Global Fund to Fight AIDS, Tuberculosis, and Malaria
IDU	Injecting Drug User
MDG	Millennium Development Goals
M&E	Monitoring and Evaluation
MSM	Men Who Have Sex with Men
PEPFAR	U.S. President's Emergency Plan for AIDS Relief
PLWHA	People Living with HIV/AIDS
PMTCT	Prevention of Mother-to-Child HIV transmission

PPP	Public-Private Partnership
UNAIDS	Joint United Nations Programme on HIV/AIDS
UNICEF	United Nations Children's Fund
USG	United States Government
WHO	World Health Organization

End Notes

[1] http://www.who.int/hiv/pub/2009progressreport/en/
[2] http://data.unaids.org/pub/Report/2009/JC1681_what_countries_need_en.pdf, p 8
[3] Ibid, p 3
[4] http://www.kff.org/hivaids/upload/7347-052.pdf
[5] Ibid
[6] http://data.unaids.org/pub/GlobalReport/2008/jc1510_2008 global report pp211 234_en.pdf
[7] http://data.unaids.org/pub/FactSheet/2009/20091124_FS_SSA
[8] Ibid
[9] http://data.unaids.org/pub/FactSheet/2009/20091124_FS_caribbean_en.pdf
[10] http://data.unaids.org/pub/Report/2009/2009_epidemic p. 37
[11]   http://www.ifc.org/ifcext/healthinafrica.nsf/AttachmentsByTitle/IFC_HealthinAfrica_Sec1/$FILE/IFC_
   HealthinAfrica_Sec1.pdf, p 5,6
[12] Ibid, p 9

In: Global HIV/AIDS Threat and the U.S. Response
Editor: David R. Carmody

ISBN: 978-1-61324-568-2
© 2011 Nova Science Publishers, Inc.

Chapter 5

EFFORTS TO ALIGN PROGRAMS WITH PARTNER COUNTRIES' HIV/AIDS STRATEGIES AND PROMOTE PARTNER COUNTRY OWNERSHIP

United States Government Accountability Office

WHY GAO DID THIS STUDY

The President's Emergency Plan for AIDS Relief (PEPFAR), reauthorized at $48 billion for fiscal years 2009 through 2013, supports HIV/AIDS prevention, treatment, and care services overseas. The reauthorizing legislation, as well as other key documents and PEPFAR guidance, endorses the alignment of PEPFAR activities with partner country HIV/AIDS strategies and the promotion of partner country ownership of U.S.-supported HIV/AIDS programs. This report, responding to a legislative directive, (1) examines alignment of PEPFAR programs with partner countries' HIV/AIDS strategies and (2) describes several challenges related to alignment or promotion of country ownership. GAO analyzed PEPFAR planning documents and national strategies for four countries—Cambodia, Malawi, Uganda, and Vietnam—selected to represent factors such as diversity of funding levels and geographic location. GAO also reviewed documents and reports by the U.S. government, research institutions, and international organizations and interviewed PEPFAR officials and other stakeholders in headquarters and the four countries.

WHAT GAO RECOMMENDS

GAO recommends that the Secretary of State direct OGAC to develop and disseminate a methodology for establishing baseline measures of country ownership prior to implementing partnership frameworks. OGAC concurred with this recommendation.

WHY GAO FOUND

PEPFAR activities are generally aligned with partner countries' national HIV/AIDS strategies. GAO's analysis of PEPFAR planning documents and national HIV/AIDS strategies, as well as discussions with PEPFAR officials in the four countries GAO visited, showed overall alignment between PEPFAR activities and the national strategy goals. In addition, statements by global and country-level PEPFAR stakeholders indicate that PEPFAR activities support the achievement of partner countries' national strategy goals. PEPFAR officials noted that a number of factors may influence the degree to which PEPFAR activities align with national strategy goals, including the activities of other donors, the size of the PEPFAR program, and policy restrictions. PEPFAR may also support activities not mentioned in the national HIV/AIDS strategies but that are addressed in relevant sector- or program-specific strategies. PEPFAR officials reported various efforts to help ensure that PEPFAR activities support the achievement of national strategy goals, including assisting in developing national strategies, participating in formal and informal communication and coordination meetings, engaging regularly with partner country governments during the annual planning process, and developing a new HIV/AIDS agreement, known as a partnership framework, between PEPFAR and partner country governments.

PEPFAR stakeholders highlighted several challenges related to aligning PEPFAR programs with national HIV/AIDS strategies or promoting country ownership of U.S.-supported HIV/AIDS programs. First, PEPFAR indicators, including indicator definitions and timeframes, sometimes differ from those used by partner countries and other international donors. Second, gaps may exist in the sharing of PEPFAR information with partner country governments and other donors. Third, limitations in country leadership and capacity, such as lack of technical expertise to develop strategies and manage programs, affect country teams' ability to ensure that PEPFAR activities support achievement of national strategy goals. Fourth, Office of the U.S. Global AIDS Coordinator (OGAC) guidance to country teams regarding development of partnership frameworks does not include indicators for establishing baseline measures of country ownership prior to implementation of partnership frameworks. Without baseline measures, country teams may have limited ability to measure the frameworks' impact and make needed adjustments.

ABBREVIATIONS

2008 Leadership Act	Tom Lantos and Henry J. Hyde United States Global Leadership Against HIV/AIDS, Tuberculosis, and Malaria Reauthorization Act of 2008
CDC	Centers for Disease Control and Prevention
COP	country operational plan
HHS	U.S. Department of Health and Human Services
IOM	Institute of Medicine
OGAC	Office of the U.S. Global AIDS Coordinator
Paris Declaration	Paris Declaration on Aid Effectiveness

PEPFAR	President's Emergency Plan for AIDS Relief
UNAIDS	Joint United Nations Programme on HIV/AIDS
UNDP	United Nations Development Programme
UNGASS	United Nations General Assembly Special Session on HIV/AIDS
USAID	U.S. Agency for International Development

September 20, 2010

Congressional Committees

In 2008, approximately 2 million people worldwide died of HIV-related causes and an estimated 2.7 million people were newly infected with HIV. The first 5-year phase of the President's Emergency Plan for AIDS Relief (PEPFAR) was authorized by Congress in 2003 at $3 billion for each of 5 fiscal years.[1] In July 2008, Congress passed the Tom Lantos and Henry J. Hyde United States Global Leadership Against HIV/AIDS, Tuberculosis, and Malaria Reauthorization Act of 2008 (2008 Leadership Act),[2] authorizing PEPFAR appropriations of $48 billion through fiscal year 2013 and strengthening the U.S. government's efforts to combat the global HIV/AIDS pandemic and other diseases. The U.S. government reported that in 2009, PEPFAR directly supported treatment for more than 2.4 million patients with HIV/AIDS and care and support for more than 11 million people affected by the disease. Although PEPFAR initially targeted 15 countries, known as focus countries, since its establishment PEPFAR has made significant investments in more than 30 partner countries and regions.

U.S. policy for combating global HIV/AIDS emphasizes the alignment, or harmonization, of PEPFAR programs with the countries' HIV/AIDS strategies and the promotion of partner country ownership of U.S.-supported HIV/AIDS programs. The 2008 Leadership Act, among its other purposes and findings, endorses the principles of harmonization and coordination to combat HIV/AIDS and cites improving harmonization of U.S. efforts with national strategies of partner governments and other public and private entities as an element in strengthening and enhancing U.S. leadership and the effectiveness of the United States response to HIV/AIDS. The Paris Declaration on Aid Effectiveness (Paris Declaration), which the U.S. government signed in 2005, calls on developed and developing countries to take steps to improve aid effectiveness, such as by increasing alignment of foreign assistance programs with partner countries' priorities, strategies, and procedures.[3] In addition, PEPFAR's new 5-year strategy, released in December 2009,[4] and other PEPFAR guidance highlight the principles of the Paris Declaration and reaffirm the U.S. government's commitment to support partner country ownership of the programs, in part by aligning PEPFAR with national HIV/AIDS strategies and programs.

In response to a directive in the 2008 Leadership Act,[5] this report (1) examines alignment[6] of PEPFAR programs with partner countries' HIV/AIDS strategies and (2) describes several challenges related to alignment of PEPFAR programs with the national strategies or promotion of partner country ownership.[7]

We analyzed U.S. agency documents and relevant studies and interviewed PEPFAR stakeholders (i.e., PEPFAR officials, representatives of partner government ministries,

HIV/AIDS donors, and PEPFAR implementing partners). We reviewed the 2008 Leadership Act, PEPFAR guidance, and the Paris Declaration to define alignment and to identify criteria for examining alignment of PEPFAR programs with partner countries' HIV/AIDS strategies. We interviewed PEPFAR officials in Washington, D.C., and Atlanta, Georgia, regarding their processes for developing PEPFAR plans and efforts to align PEPFAR programs with country strategies. In addition, we interviewed PEPFAR stakeholders in Cambodia, Malawi, Uganda, and Vietnam regarding alignment of goals and objectives, program activities, and indicators. To select the four countries we considered a number of factors including funding levels, geographic diversity, and whether or not the country was designated a focus country during the first phase of PEPFAR. To examine alignment of PEPFAR activities with national HIV/AIDS strategies, we analyzed key PEPFAR and national strategy documents for these four countries. Specifically, we reviewed the goals and objectives outlined in each country's national multisectoral HIV/AIDS strategy and compared this information with the activities and programs laid out in key sections of corresponding PEPFAR documents for each country. In addition, in our visits to the four countries, we discussed our analysis with PEPFAR officials to identify reasons for identified areas of divergence between the national strategies and PEPFAR documents. To identify PEPFAR alignment efforts as well as challenges related to alignment and promotion of country ownership, we reviewed the PEPFAR 5-year strategy, prior GAO reports, a relevant study by the Institute of Medicine, and the results of our interviews with PEPFAR stakeholders. (See app. I for further details of our scope and methodology.)

We conducted this performance audit from July 2009 to September 2010 in accordance with generally accepted government auditing standards. Those standards require that we plan and perform the audit to obtain sufficient, appropriate evidence to provide a reasonable basis for our findings and conclusions based on our audit objectives. We believe that the evidence we obtained provides a reasonable basis for our findings and conclusions based on our audit objectives.

BACKGROUND

PEPFAR Leadership and Implementation

The Department of State's Office of the U.S. Global AIDS Coordinator (OGAC) establishes overall PEPFAR policy and program strategies, coordinates PEPFAR programs, and allocates resources to several U.S. agencies to implement PEPFAR activities. These agencies (referred to in this report as implementing agencies) include, among others, the U.S. Agency for International Development (USAID) and the U.S. Department of Health and Human Services' (HHS) Centers for Disease Control and Prevention (CDC).[8] OGAC coordinates U.S. government implementing agencies and resources, establishes policy and guidance for the PEPFAR program, and is responsible for allocating resources to implementing agencies. OGAC executes its coordinating role in part by providing implementing agencies, both in the United States and in PEPFAR countries, annual guidance on reporting program results, and guidance on planning. In addition, OGAC collaborates with implementing agency officials through technical working groups on a range of issues. OGAC also disseminates weekly updates to implementing agency staff in PEPFAR countries regarding topics such as deadlines and changes to official guidance. USAID and CDC, which oversee most PEPFAR-funded programs, are among PEPFAR's primary implementing agencies. Of almost $16.5 billion obligated for HIV/AIDS activities in fiscal years 2004 through 2009, $9.6 billion was obligated by USAID and $6.4 billion was obligated by HHS.

In each partner country, teams of implementing agency officials (PEPFAR country teams) jointly develop country operational plans (COP) for use in coordinating, planning, reporting, and funding PEPFAR programs. The COP is the vehicle for documenting annual investments in HIV/AIDS, and serves as the basis for approving, allocating, tracking, and notifying Congress of budgets and targets.

U.S. Policy Documents Endorsing PEPFAR Alignment or Country Ownership

- *2008 Leadership Act.* The 2008 Leadership Act, PEPFAR's reauthorizing legislation, cites improving harmonization of U.S. efforts with national strategies of partner governments and other public and private entities as an element in strengthening and enhancing United States leadership and the effectiveness of the U.S. response to HIV/AIDS.[9] The act requires the President to report to Congress on OGAC's strategy.[10] The act specifies that the report must discuss many elements of the strategy including a description of the strategy to promote harmonization of U.S. assistance with that of other international, national, and private actors; and to address existing challenges in harmonization and alignment.[11] The act also requires the President to report on efforts to improve harmonization, in terms of relevant executive branch agencies, coordination with other public and private entities, and coordination with partner countries' national strategic plans.[12]
- *Paris Declaration.* In 2005, 133 countries and territories, including the United States, and 28 participating international organizations, endorsed the Paris Declaration on Aid Effectiveness, an international agreement committing countries to increase efforts in supporting country ownership, harmonization, alignment, results, and mutual accountability.[13] Specifically, donors committed to taking a number of steps to implement the principles of the Paris Declaration: to respect partner country leadership and help strengthen their capacity to exercise it; base support on national strategies; implement common arrangements for reporting to partner governments on donor activities and aid flows; harmonize monitoring and reporting requirements; and provide timely, transparent, and comprehensive information on aid flows to enable partner authorities to present comprehensive budget reports to their legislatures and citizens.
- *Three Ones.* In 2004, key donors, including the United States, reaffirmed their commitment to strengthening national HIV/AIDS responses led by the affected countries themselves and endorsed the "Three Ones" principles. These principles aim to achieve the most effective and efficient use of resources and greater collaboration among donors in order to avoid duplication and fragmentation. Specifically, the donors agreed to base support on one HIV/AIDS action framework that provides the

basis for coordinating the work of all partners, one national AIDS coordinating authority with a broad multisectoral mandate, and one country-level monitoring and evaluation system in each country.

- *PEPFAR 5-year strategy.* PEPFAR's updated 5-year strategy, released in 2009 as mandated by the 2008 Leadership Act,[14] highlights alignment with national strategies as a key component of promoting sustainability of U.S.-supported HIV/AIDS efforts through partner country ownership. In the first 5 years of the program, PEPFAR focused on establishing and scaling up prevention, care, and treatment programs. During the second 5-year phase, PEPFAR will focus on transitioning from an emergency response to promotion of sustainable country programs. PEPFAR's emphasis on country ownership includes ensuring that the services PEPFAR supports are aligned with the national plans of partner governments and integrated with existing health care delivery systems. The new 5-year strategy acknowledges that during the first phase of PEPFAR, PEPFAR implementation did not always fully complement existing national structures and some PEPFAR programs and services were established apart from existing health care delivery systems. The new strategy affirms the principles of the Paris Declaration and states that PEPFAR is working with its multilateral and bilateral partners to align responses and support countries in achieving their nationally defined HIV/AIDS goals.

PEPFAR Partnership Frameworks

The Leadership Act authorized the U.S. government to establish partnership frameworks with host countries to promote a more sustainable approach to combating HIV/AIDS, characterized by strengthened country capacity, ownership, and leadership.[15] Partnership frameworks are 5-year joint strategic agreements for cooperation between the U.S. government and partner governments to combat HIV/AIDS in the partner country through technical assistance, support for service delivery, policy reform, and coordinated funding commitments.[16]

PEPFAR guidance states that the partnership framework process should involve significant collaboration with the partner government and may also include active participation from other key partners from civil society, community-based and faith-based organizations, the private sector, other bilateral and multilateral partners, and international organizations.[17] PEPFAR guidance further states that a key objective of the partnership framework is to ensure that PEPFAR programs reflect country ownership, with partner governments at the center of decision making, leadership, and management of their HIV/AIDS programs and national health systems. The expectation is that at the end of the partnership framework, in addition to achieving results in HIV/AIDS prevention, treatment, and care, partner country governments will be better positioned to assume primary responsibility for the national responses to HIV/AIDS in terms of management, strategic direction, performance monitoring, decision making, coordination, and, where possible, funding support and service delivery. The partnership framework is meant to support government coordination of different funding streams under the framework of a national strategy. The partnership framework should be fully in line with the national HIV/AIDS plan of the country and emphasize sustainable programs with increased country decision-making authority and leadership.

PEPFAR guidance defines the partnership framework as consisting of two interrelated documents, the partnership framework and the partnership framework implementation plan. The partnership framework is to focus on establishing a collaborative relationship, negotiating the overarching 5-year goals of the framework and the commitments of each party, and setting forth these agreements in a concise signed document. The partnership framework implementation plan is to include a more detailed description of the approach to supporting increased country ownership, baseline data, specific strategies for achieving the 5-year goals and objectives, and a monitoring and evaluation plan.

PEPFAR Country Operational Plans

The COP is used for planning annual U.S. investments in HIV/AIDS and approving annual U.S. bilateral HIV/AIDS funding, and it serves as the annual work plan for PEPFAR activities. The COP database, which houses all COP information submitted by PEPFAR country teams, provides information for funding review and approval and serves as the basis for congressional notification, allocation, and tracking of budget and targets. According to OGAC, PEPFAR country teams in 31 countries completed COPs for fiscal year 2010.[18] In addition three regions developed and submitted regional operational plans for fiscal year 2010: Caribbean, Central America, and Central Asia.

The COP development process involves interagency coordination as well as consultation with other PEPFAR stakeholders. The U.S. Ambassador leads the development of COPs, which are created through a collaborative process involving PEPFAR country teams. The COP development process also involves collaboration with country and international partners in an annual review and planning process. According to PEPFAR COP guidance, developing an annual COP provides an opportunity to bring the U.S. country team together with partner government authorities, multilateral development partners, and civil society as an essential aspect of effective planning, leveraging resources, and fostering sustainability of programs. The draft COPs are ultimately reviewed by interagency headquarters teams, which make recommendations to OGAC regarding final review and approval.

PEPFAR 2010 COP guidance notes that PEPFAR programs should be fully in keeping with developing countries' national strategies and that PEPFAR country teams should identify areas of partner countries' national HIV/AIDS programs for U.S. government investment and support.[19] The guidance also states that the U.S. government is firmly committed to the principles of alignment with national programs, including alignment with other international partners.

National HIV/AIDS Strategies

At the 2001 United Nations General Assembly Special Session on HIV/AIDS (UNGASS), member countries committed to developing multisectoral HIV/AIDS strategies and finance plans. In our four case study countries—Cambodia, Malawi, Uganda, and Vietnam—the multisectoral strategy serves as a multiyear broad outline of its HIV/AIDS prevention, treatment, and care objectives.[20] While a national commission may be the lead coordinating authority for HIV/AIDS policy and programs, the development and implementation of such a strategy can also involve many government ministries and offices. Additional strategy documents, such as sector-specific strategies and HIV program-specific strategies or action plans can also provide further guidance for national programs to combat HIV/AIDS (see table 1 for information on national HIV/AIDS strategies in four countries). Other government ministries and agencies, such as the Ministry of Health, may also be charged with implementing sector- or program-specific strategies and programs.

Table 1. National HIV/AIDS Strategies in Cambodia, Malawi, Uganda, and Vietnam

	Cambodia	Malawi	Uganda	Vietnam
Name of main national strategy and dates covered	Revised National Strategic Plan II for a Comprehensive and Multi-Sectoral Response to HIV/AIDS, 2008-2010	Malawi HIV and AIDS Extended National Action Framework (2010-2012)	National HIV and AIDS Strategic Plan, 2007/8-2011/12	National Strategy on HIV/AIDS Prevention and Control in Viet-nam Until 2010 With a Vision to 2020
Lead coordinating multisectoral ministry or entity	National AIDS Authority	National AIDS Commission	Uganda AIDS Commission	National Committee for AIDS, Drugs and Prostitution Prevention and Control
Examples of other responsible ministries	Ministry of Health; Ministry of the Interior; Ministry of Social Affairs, Veterans and Youth Rehabilitation; Ministry of Education; Ministry of Women's Affairs; Ministry of Labour and Vocational Training	Ministry of Health and Population; Ministry of Gender, Child Development and Community Development; Ministry of Local Govern-ment and Rural Development; Ministry of Nati-onal Defense; Ministry of Info-rmation and Civic Education	Ministry of Health; Ministry of Finance, Planning and Economic Development; Ministry of Gender, Labour and Social Development; Ministry of Education and Sports	Ministry of Public Security; Ministry of Labor, War Invalids and Social Affairs; Ministry of Health; Standing Board of thePresidium of the Vietnam Fatherland Front Central Committee
Examples of sector- or program-specific strategies or other documents	Strategic Plan for HIV/AIDS and STD Prevention and Care in Health Sector; National Strategic Plan toPrevent and Control HIV Transmission among Entertainment Workers, Their Clients and Partners; Medical Laboratory Services Strategic Plan	National Operational Plan; Integrated Annual Work Plans; National Monitoring and Evaluation Framework; Malawi Government Development Strategy	National Priority Action Plan; National Health Policy and the Health Sector Strategic Plans; National Policy on Mainstreaming HIV&AIDS; Road Map to Accelerating HIV Prevention 2008; President's Initiative on AIDS Strategy for Communication to Youth	Directive 54: Strengthening the Leadership in HIV/AIDS Prevention and Control in New Situation; The Law on the Prevention and Control of HIV/AIDS; Vietnam's Comprehensive Poverty Reduction andGrowth Strategy

Source: PEPFAR country team officials and the national multisectoral strategy documents from Cambodia, Malawi, Uganda, and Vietnam.

PEPFAR PROGRAMS GENERALLY SUPPORT PARTNER COUNTRIES' NATIONAL HIV/AIDS STRATEGIES

PEPFAR activities generally support the goals laid out in partner countries' national HIV/AIDS strategies. Our analysis of PEPFAR documents and national strategies and discussions with PEPFAR country teams in the four countries we visited showed overall alignment between PEPFAR activities and the national strategy goals. In addition, PEPFAR officials—including officials at OGAC, USAID, and CDC in headquarters and in four countries—as well as partner government ministry officials, other HIV/AIDS donors, and civil society representatives whom we interviewed also said that PEPFAR activities generally support the goals and objectives set forth in national strategies. According to PEPFAR officials, a number of factors may influence the degree to which PEPFAR activities align with national strategy goals. As a result, PEPFAR may support activities to achieve some, but not all, goals and objectives outlined in national strategies. Conversely, PEPFAR may support activities not mentioned in the national HIV/AIDS strategy but that are addressed in relevant sector- or program-specific strategies. PEPFAR country teams have engaged in various efforts to help ensure that PEPFAR activities support the achievement of national strategy goals, including assisting in developing national strategies, participating in formal and informal communication and coordination meetings, engaging regularly with partner country governments during the COP development process, and developing new partnership frameworks.

Table 2. Alignment of 2010 COPs with National HIV/AIDS Strategies for Cambodia, Malawi, Uganda, and Vietnam

	Cambodia	Malawi	Uganda	Vietnam
Number of goals and objectives in the national strategy	44	31	25	20
Number of goals and objectives directly addressed by 2010 COP	30	22	25	18
Example of goal or objective directly addressed by PEPFAR activity description	*National strategy goal*: Increased coverage of effective prevention interventions and additional interventions developed. *PEPFAR activity*: Activities including prevention of biomedical	*National strategy goal*: To prevent mother-to- child HIV transmission. *PEPFAR activity*: Past, ongoing, and planned activities in the area of prevention of mother-to-child transmission.	*National strategy goal*: To accelerate the prevention of sexual transmission of HIV through established as well as new innovative strategies. *PEPFAR activity*: Past, ongoing, and	*National strategy goal*: To ensure effecttive HIV/AIDS surveillance and voluntary counseling and testing. *PEPFAR activity*: Activities including surveillance and delivery

Table 2. (Continued)

	Cambodia	Malawi	Uganda	Vietnam
	transmission, blood safety, prevention of sexual transmission, and prevention of mother-to-child transmission.		planned activities in the area of prevention of sexual transmission, including prevention and education services for adults, youth, and high-risk groups.	of data, counseling and testing, and laboratory infrastructure.
Number of goals and objectives partially addressed in the 2010 COP	11	9	0	2
Example of goal or objecttive partially addressed by PEPFAR activity description	*National strategy goal*: Improved understanding of the socio-economic impact of HIV/AIDS and possible interventions to mitigate impact. *PEPFAR activity*: Activities related to legal, educational, and economic support services, but no clear activities that directly address this goal.	*National strategy goal*: To promote the enforcement of legal and social rights of people living with HIV, orphans and vulnerable children, and other affected individuals. *PEPFAR activity*: Activities related to legal and social rights for certain populations, but no clear activities that address this goal.	Not applicable	*National strategy goal*: Enhancing the leadership of local administrations at all levels over HIV/AIDS prevention and control. *PEPFAR activity*: Activities related to capacity building mostly focused on civil society and health workers.
Number of goals and objectives not addressed in 2010 COP	3	0	0	0
Example of goal or objective not addressed in 2010 COP	*National strategy goal*: Increased engagement of the media and arts in the national response to HIV and AIDS. *PEPFAR activity*: No mention of related activities or goals.	Not applicable.	Not applicable.	Not applicable.

Source: GAO analysis of 2010 COPs and national HIV/AIDS strategies for Cambodia, Malawi, Uganda, and Vietnam.

PEPFAR and Country Documents and Statements by PEPFAR and HIV/AIDS Stakeholders Indicate Alignment of Program Activities with National HIV/AIDS Goals

Our analysis shows that PEPFAR activities described in the 2010 COPs for Cambodia, Malawi, Uganda, and Vietnam directly or partially address most of the goals and objectives outlined in the countries' national HIV/AIDS strategies.[21] (See table 2.)

Statements and analysis by a number of PEPFAR and HIV/AIDS stakeholders further indicate that PEPFAR program activities are aligned with partner countries' HIV/AIDS strategies. PEPFAR officials—including officials at OGAC, USAID, CDC, and HHS—and other HIV/AIDS stakeholders and experts operating at a global level,[22] as well as partner government ministry officials, other donors, civil society representatives, and PEPFAR officials in four countries told us that PEPFAR activities are aligned with the goals and objectives outlined in partner countries' national strategies and support the overall national program. Moreover, a 2007 Institute of Medicine (IOM) review of PEPFAR in the 15 focus countries also found that PEPFAR programs were generally congruent with these countries' national strategies.[23] IOM reported that partner government representatives in the 13 countries they visited generally expressed satisfaction with the level of alignment between PEPFAR and national strategies.

PEPFAR Officials Noted Several Factors Influencing Alignment of PEPFAR Activities with National Strategy Goals

Several factors may influence the degree to which PEPFAR activities align with national HIV/AIDS strategy goals, according to PEPFAR officials.

- *Other partner activities*. PEPFAR country programs are planned with consideration of other donors' and groups' activities in the countries, and therefore PEPFAR activities may not address all national strategy goals. In many PEPFAR countries a number of other bilateral and multilateral development partners also fund and implement programs to support the national program. Country team officials noted that in planning PEPFAR programs, they coordinate with other partners so that PEPFAR and partner activities will complement, rather than duplicate, one another and together support the national program. For example, the PEPFAR Malawi team explained that although the Malawi national strategy contains a goal of expanding workplace programs on HIV and AIDS in the public and private sectors and civil society, the 2010 PEPFAR Malawi COP does not include activities that directly address this goal because other donors and groups are implementing programs that address it.

- *Size of PEPFAR program*. The portion of a national strategy supported by PEPFAR activities also depends in part on the size of the PEPFAR program in that country relative to other donors' activities in the country. For example, OGAC and country team officials told us that PEPFAR is more likely to cover larger portions of the national strategy in former focus countries where PEPFAR is generally the largest donor of HIV/AIDS funds. This corresponds with our finding that in the 2010 COPs for former focus countries Uganda and Vietnam, where U.S. funding makes up a large share of the national HIV/AIDS response—75 percent in Uganda and 59 percent in Vietnam from 2004 to 2008—the activity descriptions directly address most national strategy goals and objectives. OGAC and PEPFAR country team officials also noted that in non-focus countries, PEPFAR programs may support the achievement of priority goals, rather than cover every national strategy goal. For instance, in the non-focus countries Cambodia and Malawi, where U.S. funding makes up a smaller share of the national HIV/AIDS response—47 percent in Cambodia and 22 percent in Malawi from 2004 to 2008—we found that PEPFAR activities generally supported national strategy goals by filling resource gaps and focusing on interventions in which country teams have technical expertise.

- *Policy restrictions.* PEPFAR may not support particular activities because of PEPFAR policy restrictions or other conflicts. For example, according to country team officials in Vietnam, until recently PEPFAR funds could not be used to support needle exchange programs for intravenous drug users. As a result, PEPFAR has not supported this component of Vietnam's national strategy.

PEPFAR programs also may involve activities that are not specifically addressed in the national strategy but that support national strategy goals. In the four countries we visited, PEPFAR officials, government officials, donors, and PEPFAR implementing partners generally agreed that national strategies outline broad principles, goals, and objectives rather than specific programs or activities. According to these officials, the general nature of the national strategies allows flexibility to support specific programs to achieve these goals and respond to countries' evolving HIV/AIDS epidemics. For example, according to PEPFAR officials, the Malawi PEPFAR program has prioritized male circumcision for many years as an effective means of preventing the spread of HIV, although this activity was not mentioned in Malawi's previous national strategy. However, PEPFAR officials told us that these programs support Malawi's broad goal to reduce the number of new infections. Moreover, as a result of the country team's working with the Malawi government and sharing information and data, male circumcision has since been incorporated into Malawi's most recent strategy. Similarly, in Uganda, PEPFAR supports prevention and treatment activities for a potentially high-risk target group, men who have sex with men, although Uganda's national strategy does not address prevention and treatment for this group. PEPFAR officials told us they consider these activities aligned with Uganda's high-level goal to reduce the number of new infections and treat HIV-positive patients. PEPFAR team officials in the four countries we visited told us they take into account sector- or program-specific subcomponents of national strategies— such as a protocol for prevention of mother-to-child transmission of HIV—as well as relevant epidemiological and evaluation data, all of which may be more up to date or detailed than the broad national HIV/AIDS strategy.

PEPFAR Stakeholders Reported Various Efforts to Align PEPFAR Activities with National Strategy Goals

PEPFAR country teams and other stakeholders described several means by which the country teams work to achieve alignment of PEPFAR activities with partner country HIV/AIDS goals.

- *Participation in development of national strategies.* PEPFAR country teams actively participate in the development and revision of partner countries' national HIV/AIDS strategies, according to PEPFAR officials, partner government officials, and civil society groups. When host governments are developing or reformulating their strategies, they often invite HIV/AIDS stakeholders in the country, including bilateral and multilateral donors and civil society and private sector groups, to participate in the strategy's development. As part of this process, according to PEPFAR officials in headquarters, the PEPFAR country team often participates heavily in the development of such strategies through direct advising as well as technical assistance through implementing partners. For example, the CDC officials in-country often help with surveillance activities and providing data to the host government in order to base the strategy on the most updated information on the epidemic. PEPFAR officials and other stakeholders in three of the four countries we visited also spoke about heavy PEPFAR involvement in the development of the strategies in those countries. These officials told us that PEPFAR's participation in these processes both improves the quality of the national strategy and creates buy-in among program stakeholders, ultimately enhancing PEPFAR alignment with national strategies. PEPFAR country team officials also told us that national strategy time frames may affect PEPFAR's ability to align its programs. For example, in Malawi, PEPFAR country officials were able to generate the 2010 COP based on Malawi's newly revised and updated multisectoral national strategy. Conversely, PEPFAR officials in Cambodia told us that Cambodia's outdated strategy, which was undergoing revision at the time of COP development and submission, complicated the country team's ability to base the current year COP on the dated strategy.
- *Meetings with partner governments and other stakeholders.* PEPFAR country team participation in periodic meetings with partner country government officials, other donors, and civil society organizations helps to ensure that PEPFAR program activities support national strategies, according to PEPFAR officials and other HIV/AIDS stakeholders.[24] Country team officials, partner government officials, and other donor representatives in the four countries we visited told us that PEPFAR country team officials participate in periodic advisory and technical area meetings with government officials and other donor representatives. For example, in the four countries we visited, we heard that PEPFAR officials participate in HIV/AIDS or health sector committees, which generally are led by the host government and include other relevant donors. In addition, PEPFAR officials participate in government-led technical working groups focused on specific HIV/AIDS-related areas, such as prevention of mother-to-child transmission or monitoring and evaluation.

- *Informal engagement with partner government officials.* Regular informal engagement with partner country government officials helps PEPFAR country teams to be aware of the needs and goals of the national HIV/AIDS program, according to PEPFAR country team officials. For example, the officials noted that in-country CDC staff are embedded in the Ministry of Health and thus have daily interaction with partner government officials. This daily communication helps the PEPFAR team focus on the needs of the partner government and align its activities with such needs. Country team officials also noted the importance of other regular interaction and communication between PEPFAR officials and partner government officials. For example, regular interaction with a number of ministry officials involved in the national HIV/AIDS program enables the PEPFAR team to better coordinate with the national program.

- *COP development process.* PEPFAR country teams engage with country officials and implementing partners throughout the annual COP development process, according to PEPFAR officials, partner government officials, and civil society groups. PEPFAR guidance states that developing the annual COP provides an opportunity to share information with partner government officials, which is an essential aspect of effective planning.[25] In the four countries we visited, officials from ministries including the national AIDS authority and Ministry of Health told us that they had discussed the fiscal year 2010 COP with PEPFAR officials. PEPFAR country team officials and implementing partners in the four countries also told us that the country teams share information with their implementing partners in a collaborative process during the annual COP development process. For example, in the four countries we visited, PEPFAR officials told us they convened technical working group meetings of PEPFAR, partner government, and implementing partner officials throughout the COP process. Through these technical working groups and ongoing collaboration throughout the COP development process, implementing partners are able to provide input on the PEPFAR program and alignment with national strategies.

- *Partnership framework development.* Development of partnership frameworks has had a positive effect on PEPFAR alignment and coordination with other donors, according to OGAC, USAID, and CDC officials and other PEPFAR stakeholders. OGAC officials reported in June 2010 that 24 countries and two regions had been invited to develop partnership frameworks[26] and that 7 of these countries, as well as both regions—Angola, Caribbean, Central America, Ghana, Kenya, Lesotho, Malawi, Swaziland, and Tanzania—had completed and signed a framework document.[27] PEPFAR officials—including OGAC, USAID, and CDC officials—told us that partnership framework development in these countries created a vehicle for more open dialogue among PEPFAR, the country governments, and other donors. PEPFAR officials also stated that alignment of PEPFAR activities with these countries' national HIV/AIDS strategies improved as a result of close interaction with a range of stakeholders. Likewise, during our visit to Malawi, PEPFAR and government officials, as well as other donors, noted improvement in PEPFAR alignment with national strategies as well as coordination with other donors' HIV/AIDS programs as a result of the partnership framework development process. In addition, our review of the Malawi partnership framework showed that the goals and objectives are closely aligned with those laid out in the national strategy. However, OGAC officials noted that the impact of partnership frameworks on country ownership remained to be seen. As of August 2010, Malawi had completed and signed a partnership framework implementation plan.

PEPFAR STAKEHOLDERS NOTED SEVERAL FACTORS THAT CAN HINDER PEPFAR ALIGNMENT WITH NATIONAL STRATEGIES

PEPFAR stakeholders highlighted several factors that can make it difficult to align PEPFAR activities with national HIV/AIDS strategies. First, PEPFAR indicators sometimes differ from indicators used by partner countries and other international donors.[28] Second, gaps may exist in the sharing of PEPFAR information with partner country governments and other donors. Third, lack of country leadership and capacity to develop strategies and manage programs affects PEPFAR country teams' ability to ensure that PEPFAR activities align with national strategy goals. Fourth, OGAC's guidance to PEPFAR country teams on developing partnership frameworks and implementation plans does not include indicators for measuring progress toward country ownership.

Differences between PEPFAR Indicators and National and International Indicators

Many PEPFAR stakeholders noted differences between PEPFAR performance indicators and national and international performance indicators.[29] Other PEPFAR stakeholders, including partner country officials, other donors, and PEPFAR implementing partners in the four countries we visited highlighted difficulties in harmonizing PEPFAR indicators with the national indicators, owing to variance between indicator definitions and reporting time frames used to collect and report data. For example, according to Vietnamese government officials, PEPFAR defines orphans and vulnerable children using different age groupings than the government of Vietnam. In addition, other HIV/AIDS stakeholders and experts noted that PEPFAR often relies on indicators that can be compiled to report globally but may differ from those used by individual countries. A PEPFAR official also noted that national strategy indicators may not always align with international indicators.

Moreover, PEPFAR's 5-year strategy states that PEPFAR's extensive performance reporting requirements were not always harmonized with other international indicators. The PEPFAR strategy also states that PEPFAR will support transition to a single, streamlined national monitoring and evaluation system. To address this problem, OGAC published an updated guide for indicators in August 2009, intended to increase both the inclusion of quality PEPFAR indicators and the alignment of such indicators with those of other development partners. OGAC collaborated with international donors and organizations including the Global Fund, UNAIDS, WHO, and UNICEF to align most PEPFAR-essential indicators with international standards. Specifically, OGAC is working internationally with multilateral partners to achieve a minimum core set of global reporting indicators that provides standardized data for comparison across countries and allows for aggregation at the global level. According to PEPFAR guidance, through the UNAIDS Monitoring and Evaluation Reference Group, OGAC and 18 other international multilateral and bilateral agencies have agreed on a minimum set of standardized indicators. In addition, PEPFAR will continue to work with this group on global harmonization of indicators. OGAC's updated indicator guidance also notes that a second wave of recommended indicators will be released in 2010, providing additional indicators that PEPFAR country teams may choose to monitor at a country level.

Gaps in Partner Countries' Access to PEPFAR Information

Some partner government officials told us they lack information about PEPFAR programs and funding in their country and expressed concern over this lack of access to PEPFAR data.[30] For example, government officials in Vietnam reported they do not have sufficient information on PEPFAR spending and are not able to fully account for PEPFAR funding to local civil society organizations. In addition, in one country we visited, officials from some ministries told us they had not received copies of the COP. However, according to PEPFAR officials, this may be caused by lack of information sharing within or among the partner government ministries and agencies. UNGASS[31] 2010 progress reports for the four countries we visited, which detail the progress in the national HIV/AIDS response, appear to include PEPFAR funding information, indicating that PEPFAR had shared such information with the partner governments. However, two of these countries' 2008 UNGASS progress reports included estimated or partial information on PEPFAR activities and aid flows; all four countries' reports noted difficulties in obtaining international donors' HIV/AIDS spending data. In addition, IOM reported in 2007 that other donors had expressed concern about the degree of information on PEPFAR programs that could be shared due to procurement rules.[32]

PEPFAR's 5-year strategy states that PEPFAR is committed to transparent reporting of investments and notes that opportunities exist to improve reporting mechanisms. The strategy also states that PEPFAR will work to expand publicly available data. According to COP guidance, the extent to which the information in the COP can be shared with stakeholders is limited because procurement-sensitive information must be protected to adhere to U.S. competitive acquisition and assistance practices.

Capacity Limitations in Partner Country Governments

Limited resources and partner country capacity to develop, lead, and implement the national HIV/AIDS program affects PEPFAR's ability to effectively coordinate with the host country government, according to PEPFAR officials in headquarters and in the countries we visited.[33] PEPFAR officials, as well as donors, PEPFAR implementing partners, and other HIV/AIDS stakeholders, mentioned one or more of the following challenges to engaging with partner governments: unwillingness or inability to commit resources, public corruption and financial mismanagement, and lack of technical expertise.

PEPFAR's 5-year strategy states that PEPFAR will work to assist partner governments, in part through technical assistance and mentoring, to support increases in government sustainability and partner country capacity. The strategy also notes that full transition to partner country ownership and increased financing will take longer than 5 years to achieve.

Guidance for Measuring Progress of Partnership Frameworks Does Not Include Metrics of Country Ownership

PEPFAR guidance on developing partnership frameworks and implementation plans includes detailed instructions for developing baseline assessments of partner countries' HIV/AIDS epidemics and of efforts to respond to the epidemics. For example, the guidance directs PEPFAR country teams to measure these efforts' outputs or outcomes, such as the number of newly trained healthcare workers. However, the guidance does not address the establishment of baselines, including indicators, for measuring progress toward country ownership—one of OGAC's stated goals for the frameworks.[34] In keeping with various Paris Declaration resolutions, the guidance that OGAC has provided to PEPFAR country teams for developing the frameworks describes promotion of country ownership as expanding partner government's capacity to plan, oversee, manage, deliver, and eventually finance HIV/AIDS programs. The guidance requires country teams to link partnership framework goals with partner countries' national HIV/AIDS and health strategies and states that partnership frameworks should emphasize sustainable programs with increased country decision-making authority and leadership. The guidance also specifies that the framework should outline plans to assess progress in achieving the goals agreed to in the partnership framework, including country ownership.

However, the guidance does not provide instructions for developing indicators needed to establish baseline measures of country ownership and to assess progress toward this goal. According to an OGAC official, OGAC has not yet devised an approach for developing such indicators or for measuring progress toward country ownership.[35] Moreover, developing indicators to measure aspects of country ownership, such as capacity to plan, oversee, manage, deliver, and eventually finance HIV/AIDS programs, can be—as has been recognized by development experts—a difficult and complex undertaking.[36] An OGAC official acknowledged that generating such indicators would involve a process of working with development partners and PEPFAR country teams to develop a consensus on both definitions and measurements. Prior GAO work suggests that performance reports are likely to be more useful if they provide baseline and trend data. By providing baseline and trend data—which show an agency's progress over time—the agency can give decision makers a more historical perspective within which to compare the year's performance with performance in past years.[37] PEPFAR country teams that begin implementing partnership frameworks without baseline assessments of country ownership will have limited ability to track progress and make necessary adjustments to the frameworks.

CONCLUSIONS

PEPFAR's commitment to the principles of alignment with national HIV/AIDS strategies and country ownership of U.S.-supported programs is reflected in the new 5-year PEPFAR strategy and in OGAC guidance to PEPFAR country teams. According to our analysis of PEPFAR and national strategy documents as well as interviews with multiple PEPFAR stakeholders, PEPFAR efforts to align its activities have resulted in programs that are generally supportive of partner countries' national strategy goals and objectives. In addition, the partnership frameworks that OGAC recently introduced are designed to, among other goals, enhance partner country ownership of PEPFAR programs. In particular, OGAC expects that at the conclusion of the 5-year partnership frameworks, country governments will be better positioned to assume primary responsibility for national responses to HIV/AIDS in terms of management, strategic direction, performance monitoring, decision making, coordination, and, where possible, funding support and service delivery. OGAC also expects the development of partnership frameworks to ultimately enhance alignment of PEPFAR programs with national HIV/AIDS strategies. In Malawi, PEPFAR stakeholders, including PEPFAR and partner government officials, as well as other donors, observed that the partnership framework development process improved alignment with national strategies as well as on coordination with other donors.

However, OGAC has not yet established an approach for PEPFAR country teams to use in developing indicators needed for baseline measurements of country ownership, although the development of such indicators and baselines is recognized as difficult and complex. Without these indicators and baselines, country teams that implement the frameworks may be constrained in their ability to measure progress in promoting country ownership and to make adjustments to the frameworks to enhance such progress.

RECOMMENDATION FOR EXECUTIVE ACTION

To enhance PEPFAR country teams' ability to achieve the goal of promoting partner country ownership of U.S.-supported HIV/AIDS activities, we recommend that the Secretary of State direct OGAC to develop and disseminate a methodology for establishing indicators needed for baseline measurements of country ownership prior to implementation of partnership frameworks.

List of Committees

The Honorable John Kerry
Chairman
The Honorable Richard Lugar
Ranking Member
Committee on Foreign Relations
United States Senate

The Honorable Patrick Leahy
Chairman
The Honorable Judd Gregg
Ranking Member
Subcommittee on State, Foreign Operations, and Related Programs
Committee on Appropriations
United States Senate

The Honorable Howard Berman
Chairman
The Honorable Ileana Ros-Lehtinen
Ranking Member
Committee on Foreign Affairs
House of Representatives

The Honorable Nita Lowey
Chair
The Honorable Kay Granger
Ranking Member
Subcommittee on State, Foreign Operations, and Related Programs
Committee on Appropriations
House of Representatives

APPENDIX I. SCOPE AND METHODOLOGY

In response to a directive in the 2008 Leadership Act,[38] this report (1) examines alignment[39] of the President's Emergency Plan for AIDS Relief (PEPFAR) programs with partner countries' HIV/AIDS strategies and (2) describes several challenges related to alignment of PEPFAR programs with the national strategies or promotion of partner country ownership.[40]

To identify guidance for alignment of U.S. programs to national programs and country ownership, we reviewed the Tom Lantos and Henry J. Hyde United States Global Leadership Against HIV/AIDS, Tuberculosis, and Malaria Reauthorization Act of 2008 (2008 Leadership Act); the previous and current PEPFAR 5-year strategy; the Paris Declaration on Aid Effectiveness (Paris Declaration); the "Three Ones" principles; PEPFAR partnership framework guidance; and fiscal year 2010 country operational plan (COP) guidance.

To examine the extent to which PEPFAR programs support the goals laid out in partner countries' national strategies and to identify country teams' challenges in aligning PEPFAR programs with national strategies and promoting country ownership, we performed the following:

- Interviewed PEPFAR officials, including the Office of the U.S. Global AIDS Coordinator (OGAC), Centers for Disease Control and Prevention (CDC), and U.S. Agency for International Development (USAID); and U.S. Department of Health and Human Services (HHS) officials in Washington, D.C., and Atlanta, Georgia, using a questionnaire regarding alignment of PEPFAR programs globally with national strategies at three levels: goals and objectives, program activities, and indicators.
- Interviewed representatives of other key PEPFAR stakeholders, including the Joint United Nations Programme on HIV/AIDS (UNAIDS); the Global Fund to Fight AIDS, Tuberculosis and Malaria; the Center for Global Development; and the Bill & Melinda Gates Foundation, regarding global PEPFAR alignment at these three levels.
- Analyzed U.S. agency documents, including guidance and strategy documents, and performed a literature review of other studies that examined PEPFAR alignment with national strategies. Among these studies was a 2007 Institute of Medicine (IOM) study that reviewed a number of aspects of PEPFAR implementation in all 15 focus countries, including alignment with national programs.[41] The IOM review involved discussions with PEPFAR officials and other stakeholders and an analysis of PEPFAR documents as well as field visits to 13 of the 15 countries.
- Conducted case studies in Cambodia, Malawi, Uganda, and Vietnam. This work included assessing the level of correspondence between goals and objectives laid out in the national multisectoral HIV/AIDS strategy and the 2010 PEPFAR COP for each country. During our visits to these countries, we conducted semi-structured interviews with PEPFAR country team officials, including the PEPFAR coordinator in each country as well as USAID and CDC officials. We also met with partner government officials in various ministries involved in the national HIV/AIDS program in each country. In addition, we interviewed representatives of other international donors working in HIV/AIDS and of PEPFAR implementing partners in each country. With each of these groups, we conducted semi-structured interviews regarding PEPFAR support for the national strategy at three levels: goals and objectives, program activities, and indicators.

To select the four countries for case studies, we considered a number of factors, including funding levels, geographic diversity, progress in developing partnership frameworks, and focus country status. Regarding funding levels, the four countries we selected represent both high and midrange levels of PEPFAR funding. Regarding geographic diversity, the four countries represent variations in the epidemic and programs that exist across regions, including Africa and Asia. Regarding progress in developing partnership frameworks, the four countries were at different phases, enabling us to observe the impact of the partnership framework development process on alignment. Regarding focus country status, two of the four countries we selected were focus countries during the first phase of PEPFAR, while the other two were not. Although OGAC has noted that there will no longer be a distinction between PEPFAR focus countries and non-focus countries, we theorized that differences in programming and alignment might exist between the 15 former focus countries and non-focus countries.

In evaluating alignment of PEPFAR activities with national HIV/AIDS strategies, we considered PEPFAR program activities that are supportive of the achievement of national strategy goals and objectives and generally complementary of the national HIV/AIDS program to be well aligned. Our analysis involved several steps.

1. For each of the four case study countries, we reviewed the national multisectoral HIV/AIDS strategy to identify goals and objectives. We then analyzed the technical assistance narratives, which describe the ongoing and planned activities for each PEPFAR technical area, in the fiscal year 2010 COP for each of the four countries.[42] Our analysis of the COP narratives focused on whether each objective and goal in the national strategy was fully, partially, or not addressed by activities described in the technical assistance narratives of the 2010 COP. Two of our staff independently analyzed the COP narratives to identify areas of alignment between the PEPFAR activities and the national strategy goals and objectives.

2. During our visits to the four countries, we discussed our analysis of national HIV/AIDS strategies and PEPFAR COPs with PEPFAR officials to identify reasons for identified areas of divergence between the documents. In particular, we discussed every goal and objective in the national strategy that our analysis deemed only partially or not supported by activities described in the technical assistance narratives of the COP. These conversations enabled us to identify four general reasons why the technical assistance narratives did not describe activities that fully support the particular goal or objective: (a) The goal was being supported by activities of other donors, so PEPFAR had chosen not to focus in that area. (b) The goal was generally the responsibility of the national government, or the national government was not interested in receiving PEPFAR support in that area. (c) PEPFAR policy restrictions prevented PEPFAR from supporting certain areas of the national program. (d) PEPFAR activities fully supported the goal, but owing to space limitations for COP reporting, these activities were not described in the COP or were described in a different area of the document, such as the activity descriptions. One of these four explanations by the PEPFAR team applied in each instance where we found no or partial alignment between the COP and the national strategy. We did not find any national strategy goals and objectives that were accidentally or deliberately not considered or supported by PEPFAR for reasons other than the four listed above.

3. We used our interviews with PEPFAR officials in headquarters and with other HIV/AIDS stakeholders, as well as our literature and document review, to verify and complement the results of the case study work.

We conducted this performance audit from July 2009 to September 2010 in accordance with generally accepted government auditing standards. Those standards require that we plan and perform the audit to obtain sufficient, appropriate evidence to provide a reasonable basis for our findings and conclusions based on our audit objectives. We believe that the evidence we obtained provides a reasonable basis for our findings and conclusions based on our audit objectives.

APPENDIX II. CAMBODIA CASE STUDY

Population:	14.8 million[a]
GDP per capita (PPP):	$1,900 (rank 187 out of 227)[b]
Life expectancy at birth:	63 years (rank 177 out of 224)[a]
HIV/AIDS adult prevalence rate:	0.8% (rank 56 out of 170)[c]
Number of people living with HIV/AIDS:	75,000 (rank 54 out of 165)[c]
Number of AIDS orphans:	Not available

HIV/AIDS epidemic: HIV prevalence in Cambodia is among the highest in Asia. Cambodia's HIV/AIDS epidemic is spread primarily through heterosexual transmission and revolves largely around the sex trade. A low prevalence rate in the general population masks far higher prevalence rates in certain subpopulations, such as injecting drug users, people in prostitution, men who have sex with men, karaoke hostesses, and mobile and migrant populations.

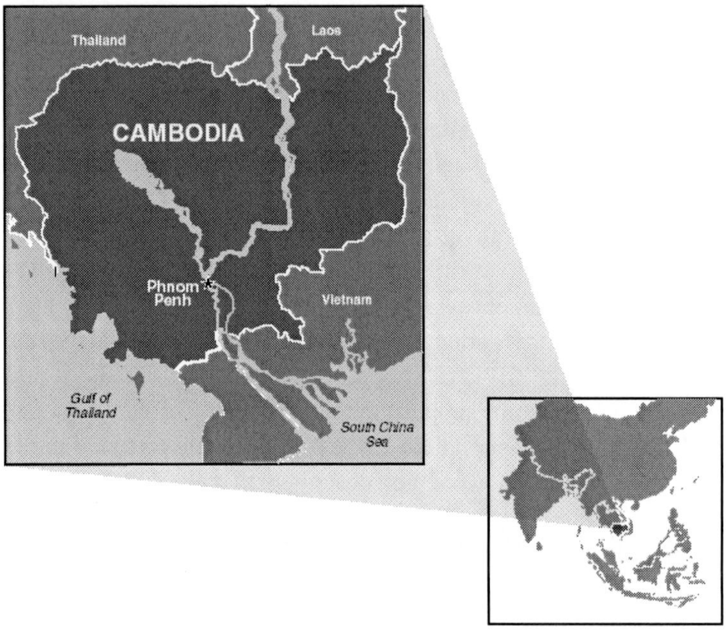

Sources: CIA World Factbook and PEPFAR. [a]Estimate as of 2010. [b]Estimate as of 2009. [c]Estimate as of 2007.

Figure 1. Cambodia Background.

National HIV/AIDS Program

Although Cambodia is one of the poorest countries in the world, HIV prevention and control efforts exerted by the Government of Cambodia and its partners have helped to reduce the spread of HIV. Cambodia is recognized as one of the few countries that has been successful in reversing the HIV epidemic, as the adult prevalence decreased from a high of 2 percent in 1998 to 0.8 percent in 2008. The Cambodia HIV/AIDS strategy—the National Strategic Plan for a Comprehensive and Multisectoral Response to HIV/AIDS 2006-2010, developed under the leadership of the National AIDS Authority—guides the national response to the epidemic. The national strategy outlines three main goals: to reduce new infections of HIV; to provide care and support to people living with and affected by HIV; and to alleviate the socioeconomic and human impact of AIDS on the individual, family, community, and society. In addition, the multisectoral strategy also lays out seven complementary strategies to (1) increase coverage of effective prevention interventions; (2) increase coverage of effective interventions for comprehensive care; (3) increase coverage of effective interventions for impact mitigation; (4) develop effective leadership by government and nongovernment sectors for implementation of the response to AIDS at central and local levels; (5) create a supportive legal and public policy environment for the AIDS response; (6) increase the availability of information for policy makers and for program planners through monitoring, evaluation, and research; and (7) enhance sustainable and equitable resource allocation for the national response to AIDS.

A large number of institutions are involved in Cambodia's national multisectoral response to HIV and AIDS. These include ministries and other government departments, such as the Ministry of Health, Ministry of Women's Affairs, Ministry of Rural Development, Ministry of Interior, and the National Center for HIV/AIDS, Dermatology, and STD. In addition, there are a number of other strategies and documents that support and elaborate on the national multisectoral strategy including, the Ministry of Interior HIV/AIDS strategy, Medical Laboratory Services National Strategic Plan, and the National Blood Transfusion Services of Cambodia Strategic Plan. Each of these successive plans and strategies has been supported by technical assistance and financial support from multilateral and bilateral donors, including the U.S. government.

HIV/AIDS Partners and Donors

In addition to the support of the U.S. government, the Cambodian HIV/AIDS program is supported by a number of other multilateral and bilateral donors. Funding from the Global Fund has comprised over 30 percent of all HIV/AIDS development assistance to Cambodia from 2004 to 2008 (see figure 2). In addition, the Global Fund has continued to scale up its funding and programs in Cambodia in recent years, and in 2009 Global Fund contributions comprised 53 percent of HIV funding in Cambodia according to PEPFAR officials. The United Kingdom has also provided significant financial support for Cambodia's national HIV/AIDS program for many years, contributing 13 percent of all HIV/AIDS development assistance in Cambodia from 2004 to 2008. In addition, other donors in HIV/AIDS in Cambodia include, Belgium, UNAIDS, UNICEF, the United Nations Development Programme (UNDP), Spain, Denmark, France and Germany.

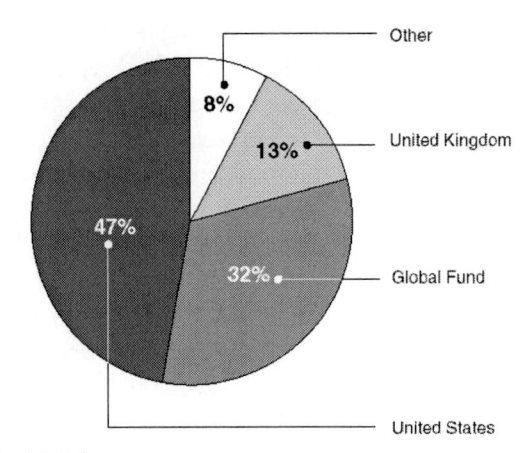

Source: GAO analysis of OECD data.

Figure 2. HIV/AIDS Development Assistance Funding for Cambodia by Donor, 2004-2008.

PEPFAR Program

PEPFAR Funding

The U.S. government has been working in HIV/AIDS in Cambodia for many years, even prior to PEPFAR, making the U.S. government one of the largest funders of HIV/AIDS programs in Cambodia dating back to the mid-1990s. Thus, while Cambodia was not a PEPFAR focus country during the first phase of PEPFAR, funding in Cambodia went from $16.8 million in 2004 to $18.5 million in 2010. As noted above, in recent years, the Global Fund has emerged as the largest funder of HIV/AIDS in Cambodia.

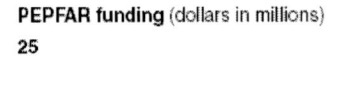

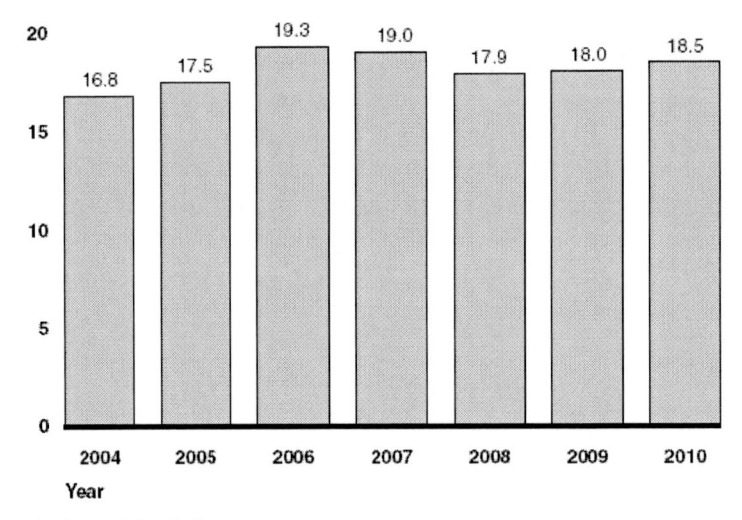

Source: GAO analysis of OGAC data.

Figure 3. PEPFAR Funding in Cambodia, Fiscal Years 2004-2010.

Table 3. Planned Allocation of PEPFAR Funding for Cambodia, by Technical Area, Fiscal Year 2010

Technical area	Funding
Prevention of Sexual Transmission	$6,167,491
Adult Care and Treatment	1,806,697
Health Systems Strengthening	1,344,900
Orphans and Vulnerable Children	1,080,471
Biomedical Prevention	1,000,000
Strategic Information	949,425
Prevention of Mother-to-Child Transmission	865,058
Counseling and Testing	573,294
Pediatric Care and Treatment	501,449
Laboratory Infrastructure	398,900
TB/HIV	382,835
Antiretroviral Drugs	0

Source: Country Operational Plan data from PEPFAR.

PEPFAR Program Information

The PEPFAR program in Cambodia supports an array of activities for HIV/AIDS prevention, treatment, and care. For example, PEPFAR focuses on peer education activities for the most at-risk population including sex workers, men who have sex with men, drug users, and clients of sex workers. PEPFAR Cambodia also supports programs such as condom social marketing, HIV counseling and testing services, prevention of mother-to-child transmission, prevention of tuberculosis and HIV co-infection, surveillance for planning, laboratory support, and blood safety. In addition, PEPFAR funds community- and clinic-based care activities such as home care, care for orphans and vulnerable children, and pediatric AIDS.

Partnership Framework

Cambodia is one of several countries with smaller PEPFAR investments and programs focused largely on technical assistance that are pursuing a strategy document instead of a partnership framework. According to PEPFAR officials in Cambodia, there are currently no plans to initiate a partnership framework in Cambodia.

APPENDIX III. MALAWI CASE STUDY

Population:	15.4 million[a]
GDP per capita (PPP):	$900 (rank 217 out of 227)[b]
Life expectancy at birth:	51 years (rank 211 out of 224)[a]
HIV/AIDS adult prevalence rate:	11.9% (rank 9 out of 170)[c]
Number of people living with HIV/AIDS:	930,000 (rank 15 out of 165)[c]
Number of AIDS orphans:	560,000[c]

HIV/AIDS epidemic: The highest HIV prevalence exists among vulnerable groups like sex workers and their clients. However, the majority of new infections occur in couples and among partners of people who have multiple concurrent partners. In addition, mother-to-child transmission is estimated to account for almost a quarter of new infections. Of the almost 1 million people who are estimated to live with HIV in Malawi, 10 percent of them are children.

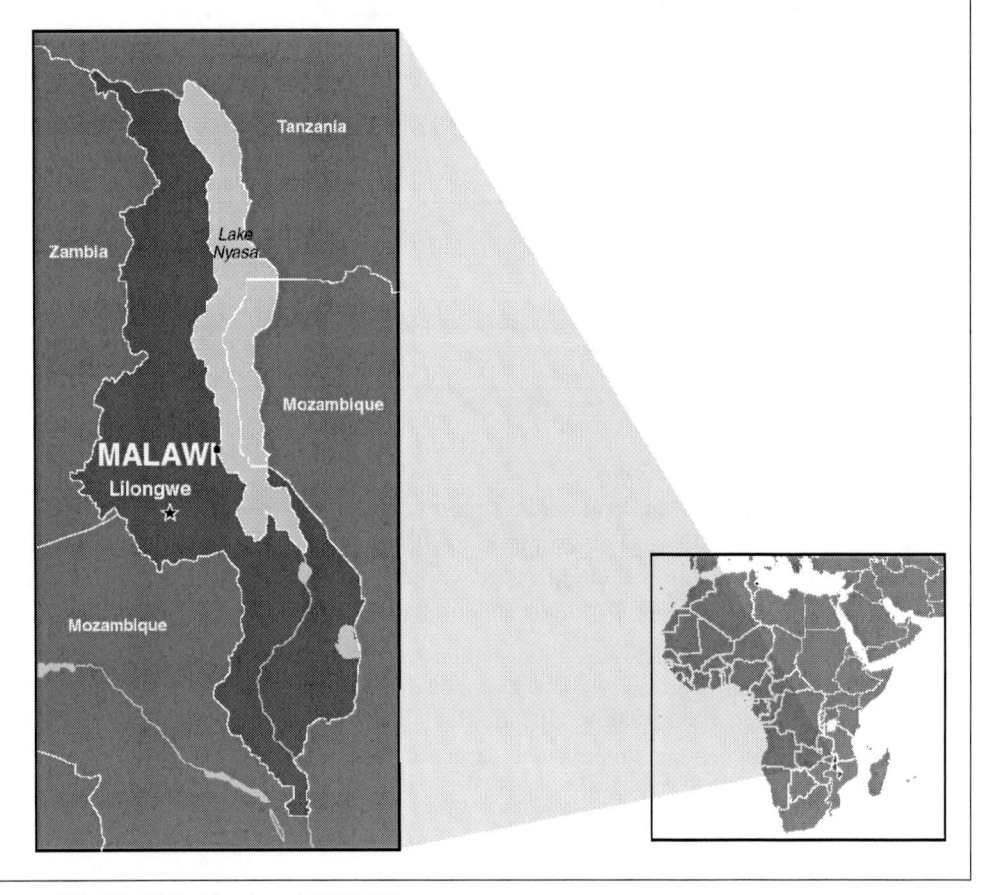

Sources: CIA World Factbook and PEPFAR.
[a] Estimate as of 2010. [b] Estimate as of 2009. [c] Estimate as of 2007.

Figure 4. Malawi Background.

National HIV/AIDS Program

According to Malawi's national strategy, the Malawi government program to address HIV/AIDS seeks to prevent the spread of HIV infections in Malawi, provide access to treatment for people living with HIV and mitigate the health, socio-economic and psychosocial impact of HIV and AIDS on individuals, families, communities, and the nation. Specifically, there are seven priority areas that drive the national response, which include prevention and behavior change; treatment, care, and support; impact mitigation; mainstreaming and decentralization; research, monitoring, and evaluation; resource mobilization and utilization; and policy and partnerships. The President leads the government HIV/AIDS efforts and the Department of Nutrition, HIV, and AIDS in the Office of the President and Cabinet is the lead government agency responsible for policy, oversight, and advocacy. In 2001, the government established the National AIDS Commission as a national coordinating authority to provide leadership and coordinate the national program. This commission is comprised of members from the private and public sector, civil society, and people living with HIV. A number of key ministries implement the national program, including the Ministry of Health, Ministry of Finance, and the Ministry of Economic Planning and Development.

The current HIV/ AIDS national strategy for Malawi covers 2010 through 2012. While the Malawi HIV/AIDS National Action Framework is the primary HIV/AIDS strategy, other Malawi government documents also comprise the complete HIV/AIDS strategy for the country. For example, other components of the national strategy include the National HIV Prevention Strategy for 2009 through 2013, integrated annual work plans, a national monitoring and evaluation framework for 2006 to 2010, as well as other frameworks, technical strategies, and guidelines.

HIV/AIDS Partners and Donors

Bilateral and Multilateral Donors in HIV/AIDS

Malawi's national HIV/AIDS program receives support from a variety of bilateral and multilateral donors in addition to PEPFAR. The Global Fund is the largest donor for HIV/AIDS programs in Malawi, spending almost $190 million on HIV programs in Malawi from 2004 to 2008, which comprised almost 40 percent of all HIV development assistance over that period (see figure 5). Other major donors in the HIV/AIDS area in Malawi include the United Kingdom, Norway, and the World Bank. The Malawi government has a funding arrangement whereby each of these donors contributes to a pooled fund managed by the National AIDS Commission.]

Civil Society and Private Sector

Civil society and private sector organizations also play a role in carrying out the national program. Civil society organizations implement activities, carry out advocacy, mobilize resources, document community practices, and support capacity-building programs. In addition, private sector organizations have the responsibility to mainstream HIV/AIDS through workplace policies and programs.

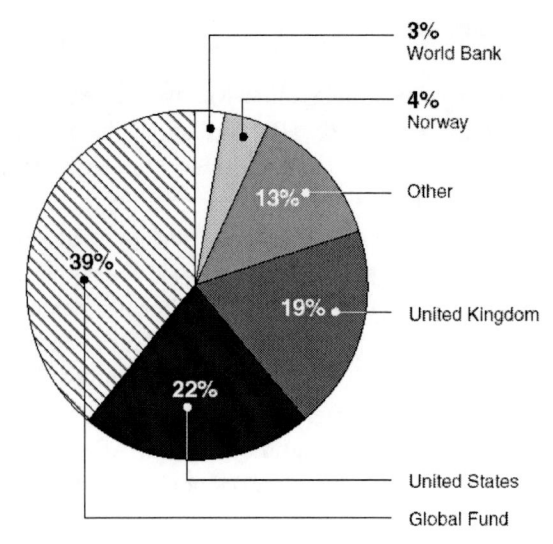

Source: GAO analysis of OECD data.

Figure 5. HIV/AIDS Development Assistance Funding for Malawi, by Donor, 2004-2008.

PEPFAR Program

PEPFAR Funding

While Malawi was not one of the original 15 PEPFAR focus countries, PEPFAR maintained a presence in Malawi with funding increasing from $15 million in 2004 to $55.3 million in 2010 (see figure 6). U.S. government development assistance for HIV/AIDS comprised 22 percent of total development assistance to Malawi for HIV/AIDS from 2004 to 2008. As noted above, the majority of the HIV/AIDS program in Malawi is funded by other donors such as the Global Fund.

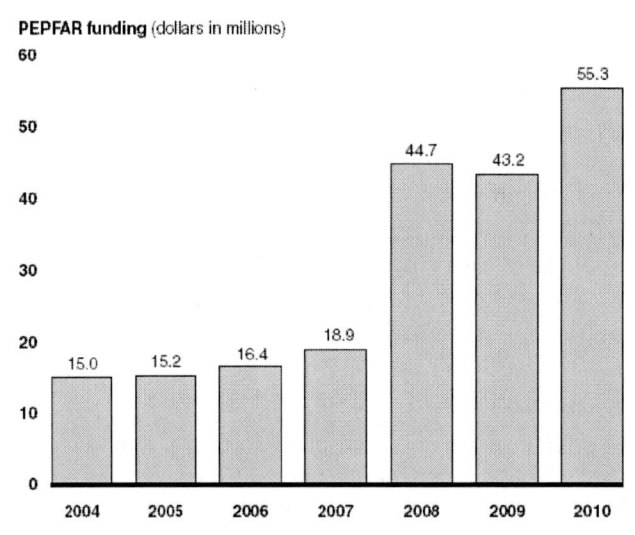

Source: GAO analysis of OGAC data.

Figure 6. PEPFAR Funding in Malawi, Fiscal Years 2004-2010.

Table 4. Planned Allocation of PEPFAR Funding for Malawi, by Technical Area, Fiscal Year 2010

Technical area	Funding
Prevention of Mother-to-Child Transmission	$12,006,294
Prevention of Sexual Transmission	8,750,481
Health Systems Strengthening	5,730,310
Orphans and Vulnerable Children	3,949,388
Adult Care and Treatment	3,845,686
Strategic Information	3,838,252
Laboratory Infrastructure	3,563,783
Counseling and Testing	3,446,036
Biomedical Prevention	2,653,168
Pediatric Care and Treatment Narrative	1,616,652
TB/HIV	912,997
Antiretroviral Drugs	$233,916

Source: Country Operational Plan data from PEPFAR.

PEPFAR Program Information

The PEPFAR program in Malawi supports interventions for HIV/AIDS prevention, treatment, and care. PEPFAR intervention strategies include strengthening care services provided by the public sector and indigenous organizations, expanding and strengthening services for orphans and vulnerable children in urban and rural areas, and building capacity to support strengthening of critical areas, including laboratory infrastructure and strategic information. According to PEPFAR officials, the Malawi PEPFAR program takes into consideration the programs and funding support provided by the other donors and focuses resources on filling gaps in the national program.

Partnership Framework

Malawi was the first country to complete a partnership framework, which was signed in May 2009. The framework lays out a 5-year strategic agreement between PEPFAR and the Malawi government, which focuses on reducing new HIV infections, improving the quality of treatment and care, mitigating the impacts of HIV/AIDS on individuals and households, and supporting systems needed to achieve these goals. Malawi signed a partnership framework implementation plan in July 2010 that provides additional detail including specific strategies for achieving the 5-year goals and objectives. According to PEPFAR officials in Malawi, additional funding was made available to Malawi for implementing this partnership framework.

The development of the partnership framework in Malawi coincided with the update and revision of the National Action Framework. According to PEPFAR and Malawi government officials, the timing of the two processes resulted in close collaboration between government officials that increased alignment of the PEPFAR program with the national program. For example, as a result of the partnership framework development process, the PEPFAR country team was invited by the Malawi government to participate in the pooled donors meetings, even though PEPFAR does not participate in the pooled funding arrangement.

APPENDIX IV. UGANDA CASE STUDY

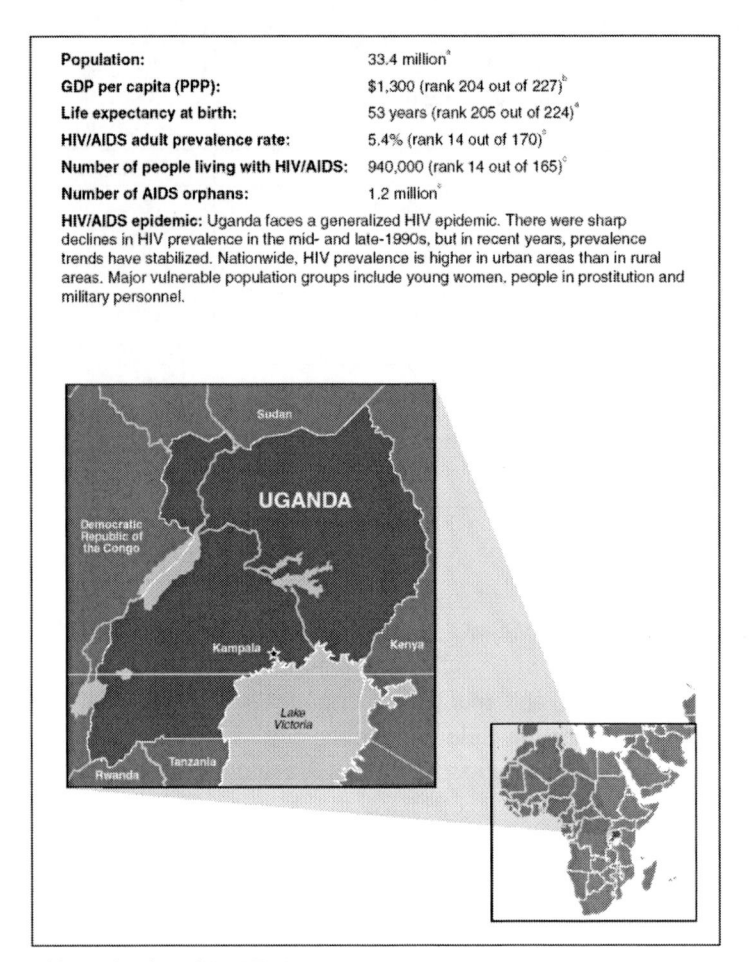

Population: 33.4 million[a]

GDP per capita (PPP): $1,300 (rank 204 out of 227)[b]

Life expectancy at birth: 53 years (rank 205 out of 224)[a]

HIV/AIDS adult prevalence rate: 5.4% (rank 14 out of 170)[b]

Number of people living with HIV/AIDS: 940,000 (rank 14 out of 165)[c]

Number of AIDS orphans: 1.2 million[c]

HIV/AIDS epidemic: Uganda faces a generalized HIV epidemic. There were sharp declines in HIV prevalence in the mid- and late-1990s, but in recent years, prevalence trends have stabilized. Nationwide, HIV prevalence is higher in urban areas than in rural areas. Major vulnerable population groups include young women, people in prostitution and military personnel.

Sources: CIA World Factbook and PEPFAR.

[a] Estimate as of 2010.

[b] Estimate as of 2009.

[c] Estimate as of 2007.

Figure 7. Uganda Background.

National HIV/AIDS Program

According to its national HIV/AIDS strategy, Uganda aims to reduce new HIV infection by 40 percent, expand social support, and provide care and treatment services to 80 percent of needy individuals by 2012. The strategy outlines four areas: prevention, care and treatment, social support, and systems strengthening. Each area sets out specific objectives and targets. For example, under the prevention area, the strategy states that Uganda will reduce mother-to-child transmission of HIV by 50 percent by 2012. Under the systems strengthening area, the strategy includes several objectives, such as effectively coordinating and managing the response at various levels. The Uganda AIDS Commission, established in 1992, coordinates the multisectoral response to the HIV/AIDS epidemic. The National AIDS Policy has yet to be approved by the Ugandan parliament. However, in addition to Uganda's National HIV&AIDS Strategic Plan 2007/8-2011/12, Uganda has developed national policies related to HIV counseling and testing, antiretroviral therapy, and orphans and other vulnerable children. The Ministries of Health; Gender, Labour, and Social Development; and Finance, Planning, and Economic Development, among others, are involved in the national multisectoral HIV/AIDS strategy. Coordinated by the Uganda AIDS Commission, these ministries, along with UNAIDS and other stakeholders, make up the Partnership Committee, which is in turn made up of various technical working groups and subcommittees.

HIV/AIDS Partners and Donors

Bilateral and Multilateral Donors

Although the United States is by far the largest bilateral HIV/AIDS program donor in Uganda, the United Kingdom, Ireland, and many other countries also contribute to Uganda's national HIV/AIDS program. In addition, the Global Fund spent over $72 million in Uganda for HIV/AIDS programs from 2004 to 2008.

Civil Society Organizations

Civil society organizations play a key role in implementing the national strategic framework. In 2007, with financial support from various development partners, the government of Uganda established a Civil Society Fund (CSF) and since has issued a number of grants to civil society organizations, including community- and faith-based organizations, and district governments to support provision of specific services by civil society groups in these areas.

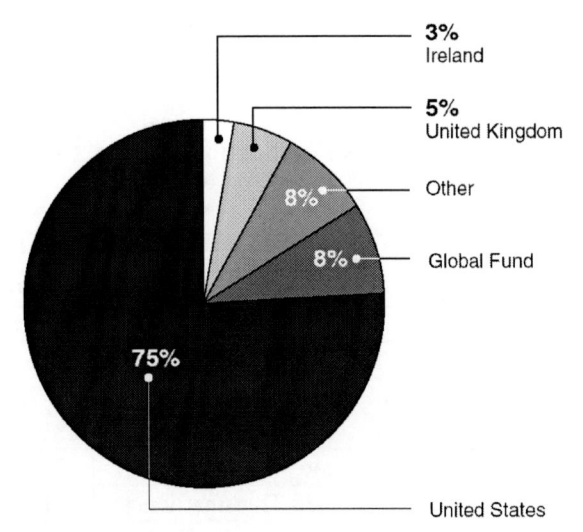

Source: GAO analysis of OECD data.
Note: Percentages may not sum to 100 due to rounding.

Figure 8. HIV/AIDS Development Assistance Funding for Uganda, by Donor, 2004-2008.

PEPFAR Program

PEPFAR Funding

Uganda was selected in 2004 as one of the original PEPFAR focus countries. As such, U.S. support for HIV/AIDS programs in Uganda increased rapidly, from about $90.8 million in 2004, to $286.3 million in 2010. As noted above, the U.S. government is the largest HIV/AIDS development partner in Uganda.

PEPFAR Program Information

PEPFAR-supported programs span a number of HIV program areas, including prevention, treatment, care, laboratory services, health systems strengthening, and strategic information. In collaboration with the government of Uganda, as of March 2009, PEPFAR supports antiretroviral treatment for more than 150,000 HIV-positive Ugandans.

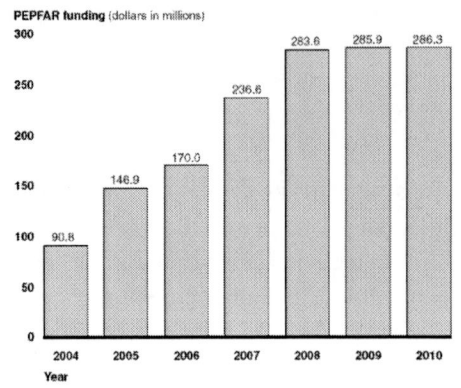

Source: GAO analysis of OGAC data.

Figure 9. PEPFAR Funding in Uganda, Fiscal Years 2004- 2010.

Table 5. Planned Allocation of PEPFAR Funding for Uganda, by Technical Area, Fiscal Year 2010

Technical area	Funding
Adult Care and Treatment	$49,294,007
Antiretroviral Drugs	45,439,658
Prevention of Sexual Transmission	28,400,685
Orphans and Vulnerable Children	25,197,969
Counseling and Testing	16,817,113
Pediatric Care and Treatment	15,365,625
Prevention of Mother-to-Child Transmission	14,910,546
Laboratory Infrastructure	13,800,894
Health Systems Strengthening	12,100,444
Strategic Information	11,891,032
Biomedical Prevention	11,624,687
TB/HIV	9,113,758

Source: Country Operational Plan data from OGAC.

Partnership Framework

The government of Uganda plans to develop new national development, health, and HIV/AIDS strategies. PEPFAR officials in Uganda indicated that these revisions create opportunities for the government of Uganda to demonstrate renewed leadership and build relationships with its development partners. In this context, PEPFAR envisions that it could pursue a Partnership Framework with Uganda.

APPENDIX V. VIETNAM CASE STUDY

Population:	89.6 million[a]
GDP per capita (PPP):	$2,900 (rank 165 out of 227)[b]
Life expectancy at birth:	72 years (rank 128 out of 224)[a]
HIV/AIDS adult prevalence rate:	0.5% (rank 73 out of 170)[c]
Number of people living with HIV/AIDS:	290,000 (rank 24 out of 165)[c]
Number of AIDS orphans:	Not available

HIV/AIDS epidemic: Vietnam has a concentrated HIV epidemic, with the highest prevalence among key populations at higher risk. These include injecting drug users with a prevalence rate of 28.6 percent, female sex workers with a prevalence rate of 4.4 percent, and men who have sex with men with a prevalence of 9 percent in Ha Noi and 5 percent in Ho Chi Minh City. Injecting drug use is a major factor driving the spread of HIV in Vietnam, posing a number of complex challenges.

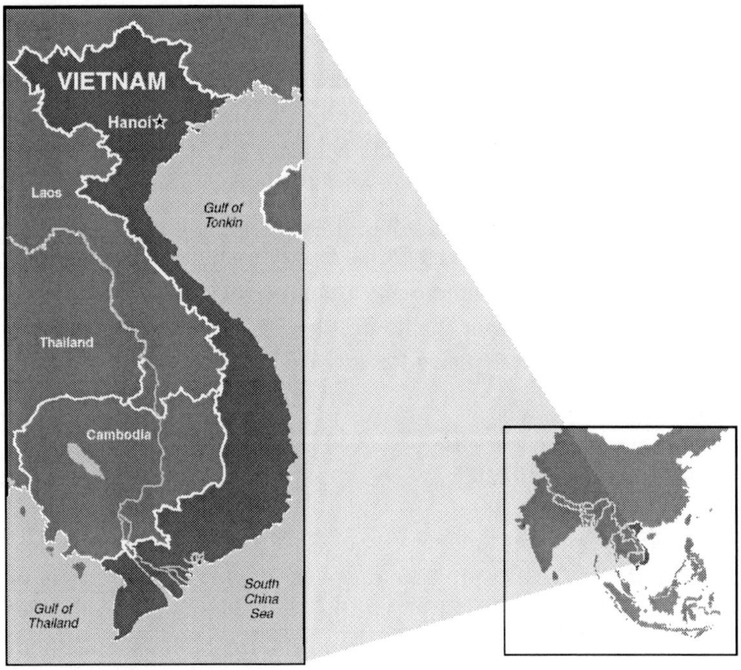

Sources: CIA World Factbook and PEPFAR.
[a] Estimate as of 2010.
[b] Estimate as of 2009.
[c] Estimate as of 2007.

Figure 10. Vietnam Background.

National HIV/AIDS Program

The Vietnam national HIV strategy, *the National Strategy on HIV/AIDS Prevention and Control in Vietnam until 2010 with a Vision to 2020*, lays out objectives and priorities for the government response to the HIV/AIDS epidemic in Vietnam. The strategy's goals are to control the HIV prevalence among the general population to below 0.3 percent by 2010 and with no further increase after 2010, and to reduce the adverse impacts of HIV on socio-economic development. In addition, the strategy also lays out a number of specific priority areas in the area of prevention, treatment and care, and HIV governance. In the HIV prevention area, the government program focuses on prevention and behavior change through information, education and communication, harm reduction targeting high-risk populations, prevention of mother-to-child transmission, management and treatment of sexually transmitted infections, and safe blood transfusion. The treatment and care elements of the strategy focus on care and support for people living with HIV and access to HIV treatment including antiretroviral drugs. The strategy highlights HIV governance issues including HIV surveillance, monitoring and evaluation, capacity building, and international cooperation enhancement. The government of Vietnam supports activities and services in each of these areas.

The National Committee for AIDS, Drugs, and Prostitution Prevention and Control is the multisectoral body leading the government HIV program. This multisectoral body is headed by a Deputy Prime Minister, and members include vice-ministers from relevant line ministries. Technical coordination of activities is delegated to the Vietnam Administration for AIDS Control within the Ministry of Health. There are also a number of other ministries and entities involved in coordinating and implementing various aspects of the national program including, the Ministry of Public Security; the Ministry of Labor, War Invalids, and Social Affairs; the Ministry of Health; the Ministry of Education and Training; the Ministry of Finance; and the Ministry of Planning and Investment. While the current multisectoral national HIV strategy for Vietnam covers 2004 to 2010 with a vision to 2020, according to the Vietnam PEPFAR country team there are a number of other strategies, documents, and laws that guide the national program including, the Law on the Prevention and Control of HIV/AIDS and Vietnam's Comprehensive Poverty Reduction and Growth Strategy.

HIV/AIDS Partners and Donors

While U.S. funding comprises the majority of HIV/AIDS development assistance funding in Vietnam, the national HIV/AIDS program receives support from a variety of other bilateral and multilateral donors as well. After PEPFAR, the United Kingdom is the largest HIV/AIDS donor in Vietnam, spending over $24 million from 2004 to 2008, which comprised 12 percent of all HIV development assistance over that period (see figure 11). The United Kingdom HIV development assistance is focused largely in the area of HIV prevention and harm reduction. In addition, the Global Fund comprised 9 percent of all HIV development assistance from 2004 to 2008, and this funding was focused in areas including prevention of mother-to-child transmission, and HIV counseling and testing. Other major donors in Vietnam include the World Bank, which funds programs in HIV prevention, harm reduction, blood safety, and care and treatment; and Germany, which funds HIV prevention activities and procures test equipment for HIV counseling and testing services. However, according to PEPFAR officials, donor support in Vietnam is decreasing because of a number of factors, including Vietnam's progress towards becoming a middle-income country.

PEPFAR Program

PEPFAR Funding

During the first phase of PEPFAR, Vietnam was classified as one of the 15 PEPFAR focus countries.[43] PEPFAR funding in Vietnam has grown from $17.7 million in 2004 to $97.8 million in 2010 (see figure 12). In addition, U.S. funding in etnam comprised most HIV/AIDS development assistance to Vietnam from 2004 to 2008.

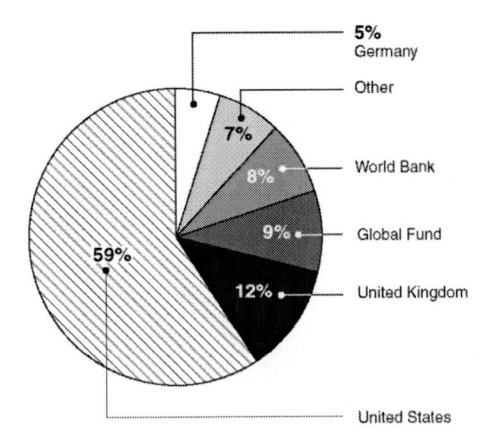

Source: GAO analysis of OECD data.

Figure 11. HIV/AIDS Development Assistance Funding for Vietnam, by Donor, 2004-2008.

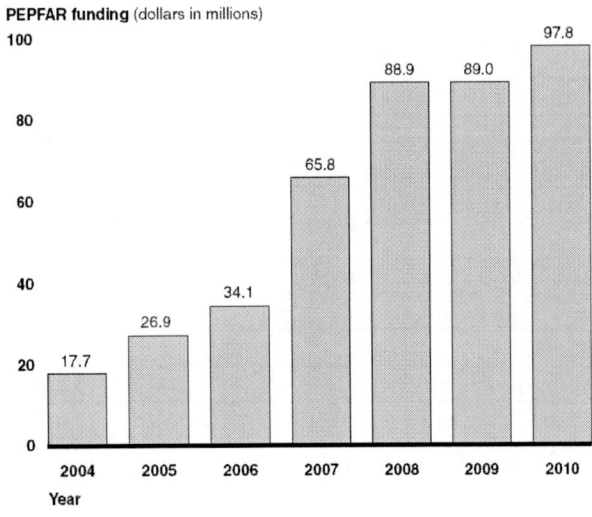

Source: GAO analysis of OGAC data.

Figure 12. PEPFAR Funding in Vietnam, Fiscal Years 2004-2010.

PEPFAR Program Information

Since 2004, the PEPFAR program has provided more than $320 million to support the delivery of comprehensive HIV/AIDS prevention, care, treatment, and support activities in Vietnam. PEPFAR activities in Vietnam have included assisting Vietnam to develop comprehensive prevention, treatment, care and support networks; supporting the government of Vietnam's efforts to reduce stigma and discrimination against people living with and affected by HIV/AIDS; training Vietnamese physicians in clinical HIV/AIDS treatment and care; assisting the Ministry of Health to develop peer outreach for at-risk populations; increasing the public health management capacity of Vietnamese government workers; assisting the Ministry of Health to develop a national HIV reference laboratory; and providing support in establishing one national surveillance and monitoring and evaluation system.

According to the Vietnam PEPFAR country team, over the next 5 years, PEPFAR will place a renewed emphasis on partnering with Vietnam to build Vietnam's national HIV/AIDS response, and continue to work together with all sectors of Vietnam as they craft strategies and programs to stop HIV/AIDS. In addition, as part of the new Global Health Initiative, PEPFAR will support Vietnam as it works to further integrate and expand access to other health care services, such as those that address tuberculosis, malaria, maternal and child health, and family planning with HIV/AIDS programs.

Partnership Framework

The Vietnam country team recently negotiated and signed a partnership framework with the Vietnam Administration for AIDS Control within the Ministry of Health. Development of the partnership framework implementation plan is currently under way, with completion scheduled for October 2010.

Table 6. Planned Allocation of PEPFAR Funding for Vietnam by, Technical Area, Fiscal Year 2010

Technical area	Funding
Adult Care and Treatment	$18,514,091
Prevention of Sexual Transmission	9,846,990
Biomedical Prevention	8,881,166
Strategic Information	6,495,182
Laboratory Infrastructure	5,637,455
Counseling and Testing	5,109,557
Prevention of Mother-to-Child Transmission	4,235,992
Health Systems Strengthening	4,027,393
Orphans and Vulnerable Children	3,552,515
TB/HIV	3,359,172
Antiretroviral Drugs	2,850,000
Pediatric Care and Treatment	2,652,078

Source: Country Operational Plan data from PEPFAR.

APPENDIX VI. COMMENTS FROM THE U.S. DEPARTMENT OF STATE, OFFICE OF THE U.S. GLOBAL AIDS COORDINATOR

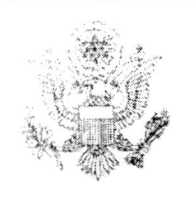

United States Department of

Chief Financial Officer

Washington, D.C. 20520

AUG 1 8 2010

Ms. Jacquelyn Williams-Bridgers
Managing Director
International Affairs and Trade
Government Accountability Office
441 G Street, N.W.
Washington, D.C. 20548-0001

Dear Ms. Williams-Bridgers:

We appreciate the opportunity to review your draft report, "PRESIDENT'S EMERGENCY PLAN FOR AIDS RELIEF: Efforts to Align Programs with Partner Countries' HIV/AIDS Strategies and Promote Partner Country Ownership," GAO Job Code 320726.

The enclosed Department of State comments are provided for incorporation with this letter as an appendix to the final report.

If you have any questions concerning this response, please contact Chantal Knight, Congressional Relations Officer, Office of the U.S. Global AIDS Coordinator at (202) 663-2579.

Sincerely,

James L. Millette

cc: GAO – David Gootnick
        S/GAC – Eric Goosby
        State/OIG – Tracy Burnett

Department of State Comments on GAO Draft Report

PRESIDENT'S EMERGENCY PLAN FOR AIDS RELIEF: Efforts to Align Programs with Partner Countries' HIV/AIDS Strategies and Promote Partner Country Ownership
(GAO-10-836, GAO Code 320726)

On behalf of the President's Emergency Plan for AIDS Relief (PEPFAR), the U.S. Departments of State (DOS) and Health and Human Services (HHS), and the U.S. Agency for International Development (USAID), I would like to express our appreciation for the opportunity to comment on the draft report from the Government Accountability Office (GAO) titled, *"President's Emergency Plan for AIDS Relief: Efforts to Align Programs with Partner Countries' HIV/AIDS Strategies and Promote Partner Country Ownership (GAO-10-836, GAO Code 320726).*

We welcome the report's conclusion that PEPFAR efforts to align its activities have resulted in programs that are generally supportive of partner countries' national strategy goals and objectives. As PEPFAR works to advance country ownership and further refine the Partnership Framework (PF) process, we also welcome the report's identification of areas in which PEPFAR alignment processes could be strengthened. As PEPFAR enters its seventh year of operations, we agree that there are still lessons to learn and significant variation among country teams' ability to ensure that PEPFAR programs support all elements of national HIV strategies. In this sense, the report is very timely, and we will take its recommendation into consideration as we move forward.

The report outlines concern that the lack of baseline measures around country ownership may limit country teams in measuring the impact of their respective PFs and making necessary adjustments. We concur with the report's recommendation that there is a need to develop and disseminate a methodology for establishing indicators needed for baseline measurements of country ownership, and that ideally, this would take place prior to implementation of the PFs. Although a number of countries have signed PFs and initiated implementation in advance of developing standardized country ownership indicators, we recognize the importance of such baselines measures for a results-driven program like PEPFAR, and will work to advance this effort in consultation with the field and as part of the broader Global Health Initiative. In the interim, we will continue to monitor implementation and progress of PEPFAR 5-year strategies in close collaboration with our in-country counterparts, with the understanding that countries will progress toward country ownership at varying paces.

In closing, we would like to again express our appreciation both for GAO's examination of this important issue and for its recommendation. We look forward to continuing to work to strengthen PEPFAR processes to ensure alignment with national strategies, wherever possible, and to promote country ownership of their national HIV response.

End Notes

[1] United States Leadership Against HIV/AIDS, Tuberculosis, and Malaria Act of 2003, Pub. L. No. 108-25, § 401, 117 Stat. 711, 745.

[2] Tom Lantos and Henry J. Hyde United States Global Leadership Against HIV/AIDS, Tuberculosis, and Malaria Reauthorization Act of 2008, Pub. L. No. 110-293, § 401, 122 Stat. 2918, 2966.

[3] Organization for Economic Co-operation and Development, *The Paris Declaration on Aid Effectiveness* (2005).

[4] *The U.S. President's Emergency Plan for AIDS Relief: Five-Year Strategy* (Washington, D.C.: 2009).

[5] Pub. L. No. 110-293, § 101(d).

[6] For the purposes of this report, alignment refers to the extent to which PEPFAR programs support the goals and objectives laid out by partner governments in their national strategy, while harmonization refers to coordination among other development partners.

[7] PEPFAR guidance describes promotion of country ownership as expanding partner governments' capacity to plan, oversee, manage, deliver, and eventually finance national HIV/AIDS programs. See *Guidance for PEPFAR Partnership Frameworks and Partnership Framework Implementation Plans*, Version 2.0 (Washington, D.C.: 2009).

[8] USAID and HHS's CDC and Health Resources and Services Administration (HRSA) are the primary PEPFAR implementing agencies. Other implementing agencies include the Departments of State, Defense, Labor, and Commerce and the Peace Corps.

[9] Pub. L. No. 110-293, § 4.

[10] Pub. L. No. 110-293, § 101(b).

[11] Pub. L. No. 110-293, § 101(b).

[12] Pub. L. No. 110-293, § 301(e).

[13] The Paris Declaration on Aid Effectiveness.

[14] Pub. L. No. 110-293, § 101.

[15] Pub. L. No. 110-293, § 301(c)(6).

[16] According to OGAC-issued guidance, partnership frameworks are not intended to be legally binding. Rather, they are intended as nonbinding joint strategic planning documents that outline the goals and objectives to be achieved and the commitments and contributions of all participating framework members. Office of the U.S. Global AIDS Coordinator, *Guidance for PEPFAR Partnership Frameworks and Partnership Framework Implementation Plans,* Version 2.0 (Sept. 14, 2009).

[17] Office of the U.S. Global AIDS Coordinator, *Guidance for PEPFAR Partnership Frameworks and Partnership Framework Implementation Plans.*

[18] The following 31 countries completed a COP for fiscal year 2010: Angola, Botswana, Cambodia, China, Côte d'Ivoire, Democratic Republic of the Congo, Dominican Republic, Ethiopia, Ghana, Guyana, Haiti, India, Indonesia, Kenya, Lesotho, Malawi, Mozambique, Namibia, Nigeria, Russia, Rwanda, South Africa, Sudan, Swaziland, Tanzania, Thailand, Uganda, Ukraine, Vietnam, Zambia, and Zimbabwe.

[19] The President's Emergency Plan for AIDS Relief (PEPFAR). Country Operational Plan (COP) Guidance: Programmatic Considerations. Fiscal Year 2010. June 29, 2009.

[20] A 2005 World Bank Operations Evaluation Department review of 21 national strategies found that most could be considered general frameworks setting fundamental principles, broad strategies, and the institutional framework, acting as a basis for subsequent operational planning. See *Review of National HIV/AIDS Strategies for Countries Participating in the World Bank's Africa Multi-Country AIDS Program (MAP),* 36194 (Washington, D.C.: 2005).

[21] See app. I for details on our methodology for analyzing the alignment of COP documents with national strategies.

[22] Some of these groups also noted that PEPFAR's creation and use of parallel mechanisms to implement programs negatively affect alignment.

[23] The 2007 IOM study of all 15 focus countries reviewed a number of aspects of PEPFAR implementation including alignment with national programs. This review involved discussions with PEPFAR officials and other stakeholders, an analysis of PEPFAR documents including COPs, congressional notifications, and annual reports, as well as field visits to 13 of the 15 countries. Institute of Medicine of the National Academies, *PEPFAR Implementation: Progress and Promise* (Washington, D.C.: 2007).

[24] In 2008, we reported that most PEPFAR country team officials (PEPFAR coordinators, and USAID and CDC officials in the 15 focus countries) who responded to GAO's survey reported collaborating with partner country representatives and major donor representatives in selecting PEPFAR interventions. In particular, 34 of 38 respondents noted that partner country technical working groups—groups organized by the partner country government that usually comprise partner country and donor representatives—were extremely or very important. In addition, 26 of 36 officials who responded to a question about country officials' participation in the selection of PEPFAR interventions reported that partner country authorities were extremely or very involved in this process. See GAO, *Global HIV/AIDS: A More Country-Based Approach Could Improve Allocation of PEPFAR Funding,* GAO-08-480 (Washington, D.C.: Apr. 2, 2008).

[25] PEPFAR guidance notes that the extent to which information in the COP can be shared with stakeholders is limited, because procurement-sensitive information must be protected to adhere to U.S. competitive acquisition and assistance practices.

[26] The following countries and regions have been invited to develop a partnership framework: Botswana, Caribbean region, Central America region, Central America region, Cote d'Ivoire, Democratic Republic of the Congo, Dominican Republic, Ethiopia, Ghana, Guyana, Haiti, India, Kenya, Lesotho, Malawi, Mozambique, Namibia, Nigeria, Rwanda, South Africa, Swaziland, Tanzania, Thailand, Uganda, Ukraine, Vietnam, and Zambia.

[27] According to OGAC officials, an additional 6 countries and one region—Cambodia, Central Asia region, China, Indonesia, Russia, Sudan, and Zimbabwe—that have smaller PEPFAR investments, with programs largely based on technical assistance rather than service delivery, are pursuing a strategy document instead of a partnership framework. The officials said that increasing country ownership and sustainability will be long-term goals of the strategy document, like the partnership framework, but it will be negotiated and signed by each government at a lower level than the framework.

[28] PEPFAR indicators are measurements used to monitor quality, coverage and effectiveness of HIV/AIDS programs and track the progress in the fight against HIV/AIDS. Indicators are intended to provide information of performance on one key or standardized element of a program. For example, to track the progress toward the legislative goal of providing treatment for at least 3 million people, PEPFAR measures the percentage of adults and children with advanced HIV infection receiving antiretroviral therapy.

[29] In 2008, we reported that 27 of 38 survey respondents (PEPFAR coordinators, USAID, and CDC officials in the 15 countries formerly known as focus countries) characterized information from the partner country's national strategy and targets as extremely or very important for setting annual targets. See GAO-08-480.

[30] According to a 2005 report by the Global Task Team on Improving AIDS Coordination Among Multilateral Institutions and International Donors, multilateral institutions and international partners did not systematically share information among themselves or with national AIDS authorities, fragmenting the national response to HIV/AIDS and constraining the ability of the partner country to identify problems. The Global Task Team recommended that multilateral and international partners regularly provide information on planned and actual commitments and disbursements, including the recipients and intended uses to national AIDS coordinating authorities and the general public.

[31] At the 2001 United Nations General Assembly Special Session on HIV/AIDS (UNGASS), the General Assembly adopted the Declaration of Commitment on HIV/AIDS. Under the Declaration, members committed to "[c]onduct national periodic reviews ... of progress achieved in realizing these commitments ... and ensure wide dissemination of the results of these reviews." A/RES/S-26/2, U.N. GAOR, 26th Special Sess., 8th plen. mtg., Annex, Agenda Item 8, U.N. Doc. A/RES/S-26/2 (2001).

[32] Institute of Medicine of the National Academies, *PEPFAR Implementation: Progress and Promise.*

[33] The Paris Declaration notes that partner country corruption and lack of transparency remain a challenge in some countries. The document also states that corruption in recipient countries inhibits donors from relying on partner country systems.

[34] PEPFAR, *Guidance for Partnership Frameworks and Partnership Framework Implementation Plans*, September 2009.

[35] The Paris Declaration states that demonstrating progress toward shared goals at the country level is critical. As such, donors and their partner countries are committed to periodically assessing, qualitatively and quantitatively, mutual progress at country level, using appropriate country-level mechanisms.

[36] At a workshop on country ownership organized as part of the Organisation for Economic Co-operation and Development (OECD) Global Forum on Development, a group of more than 30 experts from developing countries, including representatives of governments, parliaments, and a wide variety of civil society organizations, discussed the difficulty in measuring country ownership. For more information see, the OECD Development Centre, *Ownership in Practice. Informal Experts' Workshop Sèvres*, September 27-28, 2007.

[37] See GAO, *Executive Guide: Effectively Implementing the Government Performance and Results Act,* GAO/GGD-96-118 (Washington, D.C.: June 1996)

[38] Pub. L. No. 110-293, § 101(d).

[39] For the purposes of this report, alignment refers to the extent to which PEPFAR programs support the goals and objectives laid out by partner governments in their national strategy, while harmonization refers to coordination among other development partners.

[40] PEPFAR guidance describes promotion of country ownership as expanding partner governments' capacity to plan, oversee, manage, deliver, and eventually finance national HIV/AIDS programs. See *Guidance for PEPFAR Partnership Frameworks and Partnership Framework Implementation Plans*, Version 2.0 (Washington, D.C.: 2009).

[41] Institute of Medicine of the National Academies, *PEPFAR Implementation: Progress and Promise,* March 30, 2007.

[42] There are 14 PEPFAR technical areas outlined in the fiscal year 2010 COP guidance; Prevention of Mother to Child Transmission (PMTCT), Sexual Prevention, Biomedical Prevention, Adult Care and Treatment, Tuberculosis/HIV, Orphans and Vulnerable Children (OVC), Counseling and Testing, Pediatric Care and

Treatment, Antiretroviral Drugs (ARV), Laboratory Infrastructure, Strategic Information, Health Systems Strengthening, Human Resources for Health, and Gender.

[43] Vietnam was selected as the 15th focus country in 2004 and was added to the list of designated countries in 2008 by the Leadership Act. Pub. L. No. 110-293, § 102.

In: Global HIV/AIDS Threat and the U.S. Response
Editor: David R. Carmody

ISBN: 978-1-61324-568-2
© 2011 Nova Science Publishers, Inc.

Chapter 6

HIV/AIDS HEALTH PROFILE - AFRICA REGION

United States Agency for International Development

OVERALL HIV TRENDS

In 2007, UNAIDS reported that 22.5 million people in sub-Saharan Africa were living with HIV/AIDS. This figure represents nearly 68 percent of the total 33.2 million cases worldwide. New infections of HIV among children and adults in Africa in 2007 numbered 2.5 million. Nearly 6 1 percent of HIV infections in this region occur in women, a higher percentage than any part of the world. Approximately 76 percent of the 2.1 million AIDS-related deaths worldwide in 2007 occurred in sub-Saharan Africa, where AIDS is by far the most common cause of mortality, according to the UNAIDS 2007 *Epidemic Update*. In addition, the region is home to an alarming 80 percent of the world's children who have been orphaned or otherwise made vulnerabl e by HIV/AIDS.

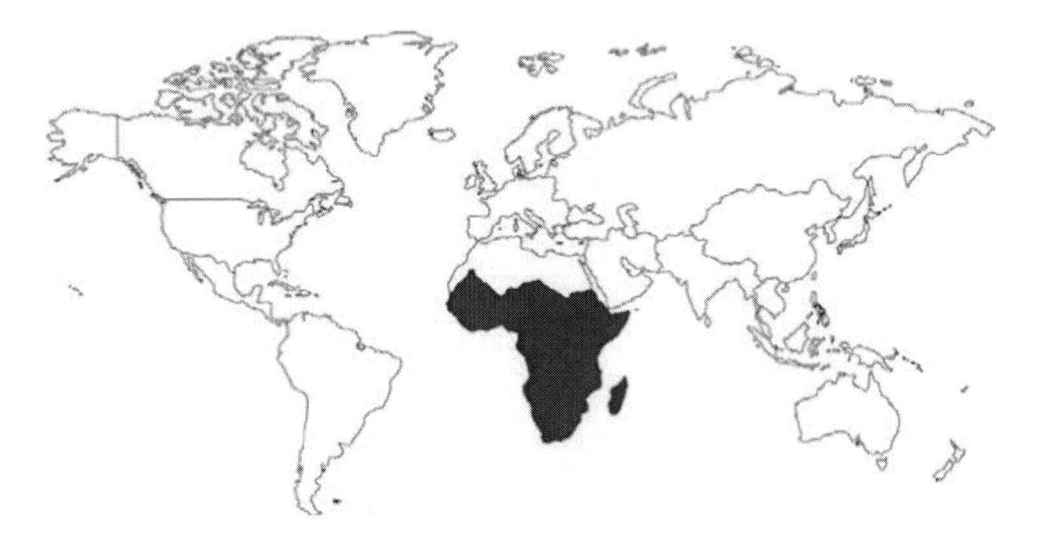

The region's HIV/AIDS epidemiological profiles vary considerably. Many of the hardest-impacted countries have generalized epidemics; others have concentrated epidemics with disease hotspots. The strategic approaches to combat this disease must be designed to respond to the disease characteristics in a particular country or region. Prevalence estimates range from less than 2 percent in the Sahel to more than 15 percent in most of southern Africa. Most countries in the region appear to have stabilized epidemics, with the number of people being newly infected with HIV roughly matching the number of people dying of AIDS- related illnesses. A recent study reported by UNAIDS that looked at data from countries with three consistent data sets from 2000 to 2005 showed that HIV prevalence declined in Kenya and Zimbabwe among young women ages 15 to 24 years who sought care at antenatal care (ANC) clinics. In both countries, a proportion of the decline may be due to a reduction in risky behaviors. Some countries, such as Burkina Faso, have experienced declines in urban areas.

As a result of unequal power relations, young women and girls in Africa are particularly vulnerable to HIV. Women are infected more often and earlier in their lives than men, and young women ages 15 to 24 are between two and six times more likely to be HIV positive than men of a similar age. Researchers believe that young women's relationships with older men contribute to their increased risk of infection. A literature review from sub-Saharan Africa revealed that 12 to 25 percent of young women's partners were 10 or more years older than they were.

The figure on the previous page shows estimated HIV/AIDS prevalence rates in sub-Saharan African countries from 2003 to 2007. Zimbabwe and Swaziland are the only sub-Saharan African countries that demonstrate a significant decline in national prevalence levels National adult prevalence in Zimbabwe was estimated at 1 8. 1 percent in 2005, down from 22.1 percent in 2003. HIV prevalence among pregnant women fell from 26 percent in 2002 to 1 8 percent in 2006. UNAIDS suggests that this trend reflects a combination of high mortality and declining HIV incidence in part due to behavior change. In Swaziland, HIV prevalence declined from 32.4 percent in 2003 to 25.9 in 2006–2007, according to the most recent data from the Swaziland Demographic and Health Survey (DHS). UNAIDS, however, indicates that the extent of these declines in Zimbabwe and Swaziland, while still significant, is not clear due to inconsistencies in the data. An important part of the decline in HIV prevalence is also attributable to high AIDS-related mortality.

Southern Africa. Southern Africa has the highest HIV prevalence rates in the world. According to UNAIDS, the subregion accounts for 35 percent of all HIV infections worldwide. National adult HIV prevalence exceeded 15 percent in seven countries in 2005 (Botswana, Lesotho, Mozambique, Namibia, South Africa, Swaziland, and Zimbabwe). South Africa has the largest number of HIV infections in the world. However, HIV infection levels might be leveling off, with prevalence among pregnant women at 30 percent in 2005 and 29 percent in 2006. Mozambique is the only country in southern Africa to demonstrate an increase in prevalence over the previous surveillance period, according to the 2005 DHS. Recent data from pregnant women using ANC services in Madagascar show the national prevalence was 0.2 percent in 2005, the lowest in southern Africa. UNAIDS data show that approximately 52 percent of all HIV-positive women 15 years and older and about 43 percent of all HIV-positive individuals less than 25 years old worldwide live in southern Africa. This has an untold effect on households, children, and communities where women are responsible for food production and child care.

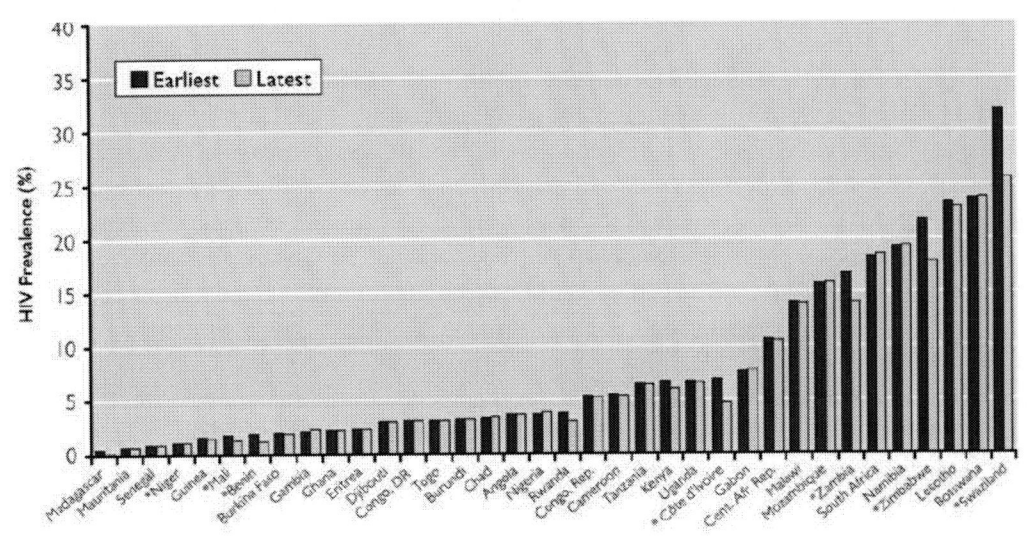

Source: UNAIDS 2006 Report on the Global AIDS Epidemic.
* Niger, Mali, Benin, Côte d'Ivoire, Zambia, Zimbabwe, and Swaziland use more recent data from 2005/06 and 2006/07 Demographic and Health Surveys.

HIV Prevalence Rate Among Adults Aged 15 to 49 for 2003–2007.

East Africa. In the countries of East Africa, HIV prevalence has either decreased or remained stable in the past several years. As in southern Africa and many other parts of the world, women in East Africa face considerably higher risk of HIV infection than men, especially at younger ages. In this region, the intensity of national epidemics varies from country to country. Uganda and Tanzania have the highest rates at 6.4 and 7 percent, respectively. Prevalence rates in Uganda declined over the past decade, but recent UNAIDS data show an overall leveling off of the prevalence rate in this decade and an apparent increase in risky sexual behavior. Since the population size is growing rapidly, a stable HIV incidence rate means that an increasing number of people acquire HIV each year. The epidemic in Rwanda appears to have declined among pregnant women in urban areas in the late 1 990s, but infection levels have subsequently stabilized. HIV prevalence is still high in the capital, Kigali. In Ethiopia, based on data collected in ANC clinics, adult HIV prevalence is more than five times higher in urban areas (10.5 percent) than in rural areas (1 .9 percent). In Kenya, HIV prevalence in pregnant women has been declining, and information from UNAIDS and the Ministry of Health indicates that national adult HIV prevalence is estimated to have fallen from 10 percent in the late 1 990s to just over 5 percent in 2006. According to UNAIDS, a recent research study reported that factors associated with this decline include a decrease in the proportion of adults with multiple sexual partners, delay in age of sexual debut among women, and an increase in condom use. In addition to these behavioral factors, increased mortality and the saturation of infection among people most at risk of HIV have also influenced the decline in prevalence. Despite this decline, Kenya continues to have a serious AIDS epidemic.

West Africa. UNAIDS data show that West Africa has the lowest HIV rates in sub-Saharan Africa. In many countries, the epidemic appears to be stabilized, although concentrated epidemics do exist. In Senegal, for example, national prevalence is less than 1 percent, yet it is as high as 30 percent among commercial sex workers in urban areas.

National adult HIV prevalence exceeds 3 percent only in Côte d'Ivoire and Nigeria and is 2 percent or lower in several other countries in the region. HIV prevalence in urban areas appeared to decline from 10 percent in 2001 to 6.9 percent in 2005. Data from the 2005 DHS show that Côte d'Ivoire has the highest adult prevalence in West Africa at 4.7 percent, yet this represents a significant decline from earlier prevalence levels of 7.0, which were based on data from UNAIDS. Significant declines in HIV prevalence among pregnant women in urban areas have been observed in Burkina Faso and Togo as well. In Ghana, prevalence data from ANC clinics ranged from 2.3 to 3.6 percent between 2000 and 2006, and, according to the 2006 DHS, HIV prevalence in Mali is also declining. UNAIDS, however, indicates that the extent of the declines is not clear due to a refined methodology that was used to develop the prevalence rate estimates. Nigeria has the largest epidemic in the subregion, with 2.9 million people living with HIV. Although the HIV prevalence is relatively low at 3.1 percent, Nigeria has the second largest HIV disease burden in the world due to its large population. UNAIDS estimates national prevalence among pregnant women varies considerably from 1 .6 percent in the west to 1 0 percent in the southeast.

Comprehensive knowledge of HIV remains low in sub-Saharan Africa and is an obstacle to reducing incidence rates. For example, approximately 2 million South Africans living with HIV do not know that they are infected, believe they are not in danger of becoming infected, and are unaware they can transmit the virus to others. Intensified efforts to increase HIV prevention among young people are also required.

The detection of extensively drug-resistant tuberculosis (XDR-TB) in sub-Saharan Africa also poses a grave threat, especially to populations with high rates of HIV and in areas where there are few health care resources. People living with HIV are particularly vulnerable to developing drug-resistant TB because of their increased susceptibility to infection and progression to active TB. Furthermore, TB is one of the main causes of death for people living with HIV. According to UNAIDS, this is particularly an issue in South Africa, where an estimated 44 percent of TB patients are also HIV-infected. Recent World Health Organization (WHO) data show that HIV prevalence in incident TB cases is also very high in other African countries, such as Zimbabwe (43 percent), Mozambique (30 percent), Tanzania (18 percent), and Kenya (52 percent). Although HIV testing for TB patients is increasing quickly in the Africa region, HIV-infected people are not typically screened for TB, though this is a relatively efficient method of case finding. There is an urgent need for improved access to TB culture and drug sensitivity testing, and the introduction of effective infection control practices in HIV care clinics to prevent the spread of TB.

Sustained progress in the response to AIDS will only be attained by intensifying HIV prevention and treatment simultaneously. Provision of antiretroviral therapy (ART) has expanded in sub-Saharan Africa. More than 1 million people were receiving ART by June 2006, a tenfold increase since December 2003. However, ART coverage varies greatly from country to country. Nigeria has the second largest number of people living with HIV in the world, but, according to UNAIDS and WHO, in 2006, only 15 percent of those in need were receiving treatment. By contrast, Botswana has almost universal coverage. In UNAIDS' view, concerted efforts for a combined prevention and treatment response could reduce the number of AIDS deaths by as much as 27 percent and the number of new infections by as much as 55 percent by 2020.

ECONOMIC AND SOCIAL IMPACT OF HIV/AIDS IN AFRICA

The HIV/AIDS epidemic is erasing decades of progress in increasing the life expectancy of the people of sub-Saharan Africa. The vast majority of people in Africa who have HIV/AIDS are between the ages of 15 and 49, and millions of adults are dying young or in early middle age. According to the World Bank 2006 publication *Disease and Mortality in Sub-Saharan Africa*, life expectancy peaked in the early 1 990s at 50 years and has since fallen by almost four years. In Swaziland, life expectancy fell from 60 years in 1997 to 3 1 .3 years in 2004. With the increase in AIDS-related mortality among 20- to 49-year-olds, adults in their most economically productive years are most affected.

The epidemic is also reversing progress in poverty reduction. AIDS tends to affect the poor more heavily than other population groups. A study in Burkina Faso, Rwanda, and Uganda reported by the United Nations Development Program has calculated that AIDS will increase the percentage of people living in extreme poverty from 45 percent in 2000 to 5 1 percent in 2015. Swaziland's Human Development Index has fallen considerably, with 69 percent of the population living below the poverty line. Economic activity and social progress are set back as more of the labor force becomes ill or dies. Agriculture is neglected or abandoned due to household illness, adding to food insecurity in many areas. In Malawi, where the agriculture workforce is expected to shrink by 14 percent by 2020, HIV/AIDS is the source of the country's falling agricultural output. In Mozambique, Botswana, Namibia, and Zimbabwe, the International Labor Organization estimates that the agricultural workforce loss could be as high as 20 percent by 2020; therefore, businesses have a stake in responding to the epidemic, which affects their workforces and can reduce markets for their goods. A study funded by the U.S. Agency for International Development (USAID) to assess the impact of AIDS on the education sector in Swaziland found that with the AIDS epidemic, 1 3,000 teachers would need to be trained during the projection period of 2003–201 1, compared with 5,093 without an epidemic.

The U.S. Government (USG) is working with the private sector in HIV prevention efforts as shown through the following examples from Zambia and Kenya. In Zambia, the USG is collaborating with the tourism industry to host a series of music events that call for social and behavioral change to reduce sexual transmission of HIV. In Kenya, the USG has partnered with the Kenya Medical Research Institute and four sugar companies to expand HIV treatment and care for approximately 60,000 people, including 1 6,000 workers, their families, and other community residents.

HIV/AIDS poses increasingly heavy demands on Africa's health systems. In Swaziland, rising morbidity is increasing patient loads at all levels. As demand for services increase, countries are losing their capacity to supply them. Providing ART to those in need in Tanzania, for example, would require the full-time services of almost half the existing health care workforce. Most health systems in Africa already face labor shortages due to worker migration to other regions in pursuit of better pay and working conditions. HIV/AIDS is now exacerbating this shortage by affecting large numbers of the remaining health care workers. Botswana, for example, lost 17 percent of its health care workforce between 1999 and 2005. In Zambia, a study of midwives found that 40 percent were HIV positive.

HIV/AIDS can have devastating effects on households. Many families lose their primary income earners, while others lose the incomes of family members forced to stay home and care for the sick. Caring for an individual with HIV/AIDS in sub-Saharan Africa can take up as much as one-third of a family's monthly income. A study conducted by the Joint Economic Aids and Poverty Program in South Africa found that it cost the country's citizens seven times more to bury a person than to care for a sick relative. Research studies show that the heaviest impact of HIV/AIDS tends to fall on widows and their family members.

According to UNAIDS and UNICEF, 80 percent of all the world's children orphaned by HIV/AIDS are in sub-Saharan Africa, more than half of whom are between the ages of 10 and 15. More than 1 1 .4 million children under the age of 1 8 in sub- Saharan Africa have lost at least one parent to HIV/AIDS. The orphan crisis is expected to worsen considerably in the coming years. Many of these children are raised by their grandparents or live in households headed by other children. As more parents die, the effect of HIV/AIDS on the region's children cannot be overstated. Many children orphaned by AIDS lose their childhood and are forced by circumstances to become producers of income or food, or caregivers for sick family members. They suffer their own increased health problems related to inadequate nutrition, housing, clothing, and basic care. They are also less able than other children to attend school regularly. A recent *Literature Review on the Impact of Education Levels on HIV/AIDS Prevalence Rates* by the World Food Program found that rising HIV rates were correlated with lower levels of education. A Zambian study from the same source found that AIDS spread twice as fast among uneducated girls.

Finally, HIV-related stigma and discrimination in sub-Saharan Africa create major barriers to preventing further infection, alleviating impact, and providing adequate care, support, and treatment. Stigma often leads to discrimination and other violations of human rights, which affect the well-being of people living with HIV. People living with HIV are denied the right to health care, work, education, and freedom of movement. Therefore, there is a need for a multisectoral response to change social and cultural beliefs and behaviors and modify policies by governments and employers.

PARTNERING FOR SUCCESS: USAID AND THE U.S. PRESIDENT'S EMERGENCY PLAN FOR AIDS RELIEF

The U.S. President's Emergency Plan for AIDS Relief (Emergency Plan/PEPFAR) is the largest commitment ever by any nation for an international health initiative dedicated to a single disease. To date, the U.S. has committed $1 8.8 billion to the fight against the global HIV/AIDS pandemic, exceeding its original commitment of $15 billion over five years.

Reauthorized on July 30, 2008, the U.S. is continuing its commitment to global AIDS in the amount of $39 billion for HIV/AIDS bilateral programs and contributions to the Global Fund to Fight AIDS, Tuberculosis and Malaria. Working in partnership with host nations, the initiative will support antiretroviral treatment for at least 3 million people, prevention of 12 million new HIV infections, and care and support for 12 million people, including 5 million orphans and vulnerable children.

The Emergency Plan encompasses all USG international HIV/AIDS activities, including those implemented by USAID. Under the Emergency Plan in Africa, USAID's staff of foreign service officers, trained physicians, epidemiologists, and public health advisors work with host governments, nongovernmental organizations (NGOs), and the private sector to provide training, technical assistance, and supplies – including pharmaceuticals – to prevent and reduce the transmission of HIV/AIDS and provide care and treatment to people living with HIV/AIDS (PLWHA). In fiscal year 2008, USAID continued efforts to prevent the spread of HIV/AIDS using several interventions:

- The ABC (Abstinence, Be faithful, correct and consistent use of Condoms) approach to preventing sexual transmission of HIV
- Research and interventions on the prevention of AIDS through male circumcision
- Prevention of further HIV transmission with PLWHA
- Prevention of mother-to-child HIV transmission (PMTCT)
- Voluntary counseling and testing (VCT)
- Injection safety and ensuring the safety of blood supplies
- Provision of therapy for concurrent illnesses and opportunistic infections, as well as palliative care
- Nutritional therapy
- Provision of ART for PLWHA
- Support for OVC

USAID is uniquely positioned to support multisectoral responses to HIV/AIDS that address the widespread impact of the disease outside the health sector. In particular, USAID is supporting cross-sector programs in areas such as agriculture, education, democracy, and trade that link to HIV/AIDS and mutually support the objective of reducing the impact of the pandemic on nations, communities, families, and individuals. Under the Emergency Plan, USAID also supports a number of international partnerships; provides staff support to the Global Fund to Fight AIDS, Tuberculosis and Malaria; and works with local coordinating committees of the Global Fund to improve implementation of the Fund programs and their complement to USG programs. Finally, USAID supports targeted research on vaccines, the development and dissemination of new technologies, new packaging and distribution mechanisms for antiretroviral (ARV) drugs, training for improved local responses to the epidemic from NGOs and faith-based organizations, and infrastructure development for appropriate clinical design and laboratory facilities.

USAID COUNTRY SUPPORT IN AFRICA

In sub-Saharan Africa, USAID support of the Emergency Plan places special emphasis on 12 focus countries: Botswana, Côte d'Ivoire, Ethiopia, Kenya, Mozambique, Namibia, Nigeria, Rwanda, South Africa, Tanzania, Uganda, and Zambia. In addition, HIV/AIDS programs are also implemented in many other countries, including Angola, Benin, the Democratic Republic of the Congo (DR Congo), Eritrea, Ghana, Guinea, Lesotho, Liberia, Madagascar, Malawi, Mali, Senegal, Sudan, Swaziland, and Zimbabwe.

Examples of USAID assistance include the following activities and interventions:

- In Ethiopia, 516,800 people received counseling and testing to detect HIV and prevent further spread of the infection.

- In Kenya, 239,600 OVC received direct care and support services.
- In South Africa, the cumulative number of HIV-positive pregnant women receiving ARV prophylaxis increased from 76,000 by the end of 2004 to 251,400 by the end of 2006, averting an estimated 47,700 infant infections.
- USAID assisted Namibia with the development of the national policy on OVC, which the Ministry of Women Affairs and Child Welfare completed and endorsed. In 2006, 88,700 children were served by an OVC program.
- In Lesotho, USAID supported an assessment of the national PMTCT program, resulting in a follow-on request for increased support to the national program. In response, USAID funded and organized a partnership to coordinate PMTCT activities with government counterparts. By the end of 2008, the partnership will provide PMTCT services in seven of 10 districts nationwide, including seven hospitals, three filter clinics, and 47 health centers.
- In Ghana, USAID supported nutrient-dense take-home food rations for 14,000 PLWHA, OVC, and their family members, and psychosocial counseling for 686 people.
- Expanded VCT services in Mali (from four centers to 169 through use of mobile services) increased the number of individuals tested for HIV by 48 percent. Mobile services improve the accessibility to HIV testing, particularly for high- risk groups.
- The Red Card Initiative in Madagascar empowered adolescent girls to say "no" to risky sexual situations. The Initiative reached 900,000 girls ages 10 to 14. More than 78,300 at-risk youth received quality counseling and reproductive health services (a 122 percent increase from the previous year) through a franchised network of private sector service providers in seven high-risk cities. One positive impact of the program was an increase in youth ages 15 to 18 who had never had sexual intercourse from 65.6 percent in 2003 to 82 percent in 2006.
- USAID supported the Swaziland National AIDS Program in HIV testing and counseling. The Agency has been at the forefront of policy, technical guidance, service delivery, and training for national HIV testing and counseling scale-up. The USG has provided substantial assistance to the rollout of Swaziland's provider-initiated counseling and testing plan while maintaining an important focus on outreach and client-initiated counseling and testing.
- USAID supported Benin in the adoption of a national law that prohibits stigma and discrimination against PLWHA.
- In the DR Congo, USAID-supported community outreach to prevent HIV reached more than 148,000 individuals. USAID also supported the promotion of condom social marketing, with 8.1 million condoms distributed in 2007 in Bukavu, Lubumbashi, and Matadi, and palliative care for more than 3,200 PLWHA.

Important Links

USAID HIV/AIDS Web site for Africa: http://www.usaid.gov/our_work/global_health For more information, see USAID's HIV/AIDS Web site: http://www.usaid.gov/our_work/ global_health/aids

In: Global HIV/AIDS Threat and the U.S. Response
Editor: David R. Carmody

ISBN: 978-1-61324-568-2
© 2011 Nova Science Publishers, Inc.

Chapter 7

HIV/AIDS HEALTH PROFILE - ASIA REGION

United States Agency for International Development

OVERALL HIV TRENDS

National HIV infection levels in Asia are low compared with those in Africa. HIV prevalence is highest in Southeast Asia, with wide variation in epidemic trends among different countries. Burma and Cambodia show declines in prevalence, but the epidem ic is growing at a particularly high rate in Indonesia (particularly in the Papua Province) and Vietnam. In East Asia, there were almost 20 percent more new HIV infections in 2007 compared with 2001. In South and Southeast Asia, the number of new HIV infection s decreased from 450,000 in 2001 to 340,000 in 2007. Even though prevalence rates may be low, the large populations of many Asian nations mean that large numbers of people have HIV infection. For the Asia region, the latest estimates show that 4 .9 million people were living with HIV in 2007, including 440,000 people who became newly infected in the past year, and that AIDS claimed approximately 300,000 lives in 2007 (UNAIDS, November 2007). In East Asia, approximately 800,000 people were living with HIV, and AIDS claimed 32,000 lives in this subregion in 2007, according to UNAIDS. As of 2005, ap proximately 52,400 people living in Central Asia were HIV positive.

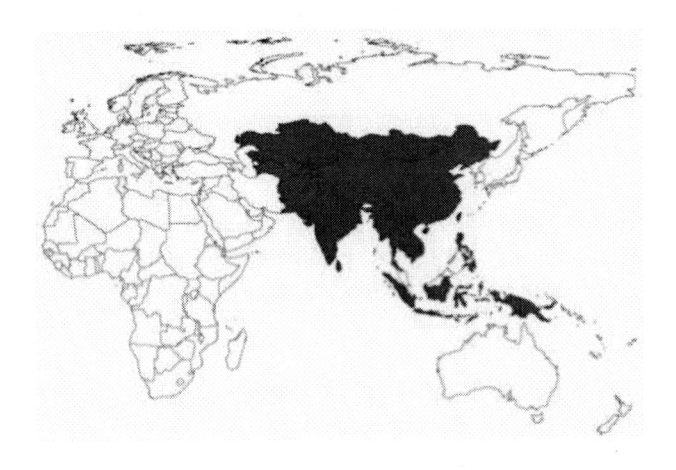

The figure below shows recent trends of HIV prevalence in selected Asian countries. Cambodia and Thailand, two countries that successfully curbed their earlier epidemics, are designing and implementing programs to reduce HIV transmission among groups who were not the central focus of previous responses, such as injecting drug users (IDUs), sex workers, and men who have sex with men (MSM). Thailand has made considerable progress providing HIV treatment to 88 percent of those who need it, according to a recent report (WHO/UNAIDS/UNICEF, *Towards Universal Access*, April 2007). In Cambodia, the national HIV prevalence has fallen to an estimated 0.6 percent among the adult (15–49 years) population in 2006, down from a peak of 2 percent in 1998.

India has a lower prevalence than Cambodia and Thailand but has significantly more people living with HIV infection, an estimated 2.5 million in 2006, according to the 2006 National Family Health Survey. However, HIV prevalence in India varies widely between states and regions. Although the majority of people living with HIV reside in four southern states (Andhra Pradesh, Karnataka, Maharashtra, and Tamil Nadu), prevalence tends to be concentrated in certain districts. HIV prevalence in southern states overall is four to five times higher than in northern states. Data from 2006 sentinel surveillance show stable or declining prevalence among pregnant women in the four southern states, but prevalence is high among sex workers and rising among IDUs and MSM in a few states. Knowledge about HIV/AIDS is limited in India, with only 84 percent of men and 61 percent of women saying they have ever heard of AIDS.

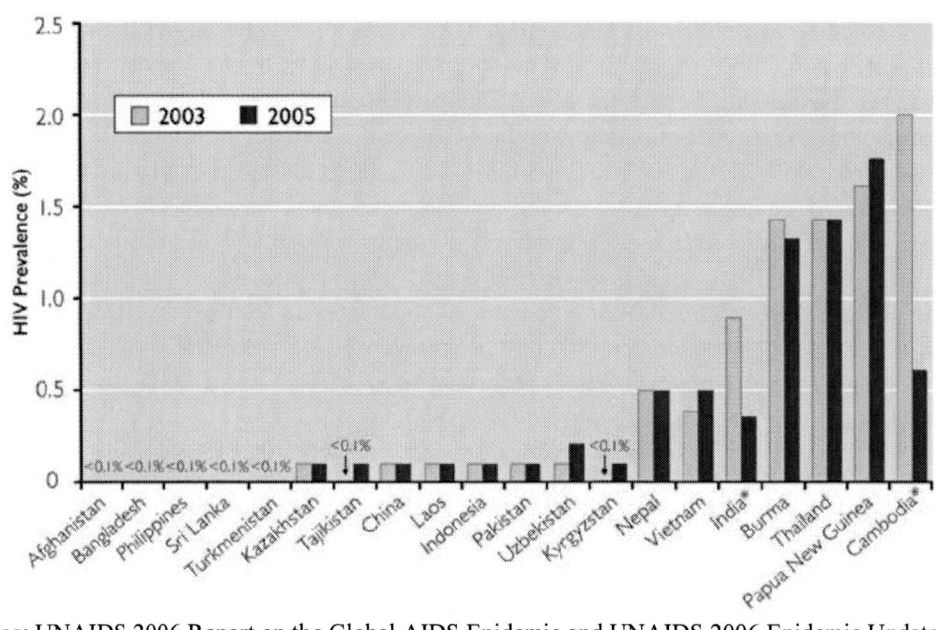

Source: UNAIDS 2006 Report on the Global AIDS Epidemic and UNAIDS 2006 Epidemic Update
*Cambodia data are from the 2005 Cambodia Demographic and Health Survey. India data are from the National Family Health Survey 2005–06. The decline in HIV prevalence observed between 2003 and 2005 in both countries is probably due to a change in the methodology used to calculate HIV prevalence.

Trends in HIV Prevalence, 2003–2005.

In Vietnam, a focus country in the U.S. President's Emergency Plan for AIDS Relief (Emergency Plan/PEPFAR), the epidemic continues to increase, with HIV having been detected in all 64 provinces and all cities. In 2005, the number of people living with AIDS reached 260,000 (twice the number in 2000), largely because of use of contaminated injecting equipment and unprotected sex with nonregular partners or sex workers. Prevalence increased from 9 percent in 1996 to 34 percent in 2005 among IDUs.

Risky behaviors (often more than one) continue to sustain serious AIDS epidemics in Asia. At the heart of many of Asia's epidemics lies the interaction between injecting drug use and unprotected sex, much of it commercial. The characteristics of transmission, such as the percentage attributed to IDUs or sex workers, vary greatly among countries. Most infections occur around corridors or areas of development and industrialization, where mobile populations, migrant workers, and sex workers are key factors in transmission.

The rate of HIV infections in the region attributed to injecting drug use is growing. In China and Indonesia, injecting drug use is the leading cause of HIV infection at 44 percent. Although prevalence is low in China and Indonesia at 0.1 percent, 650,000 and 170,000 people, respectively, are currently living with HIV/AIDS due to the large population size of the two countries. For instance, in Jakarta, more than 40 percent of IDUs tested HIV positive in 2005. In some South and Southeast Asian countries, such as Pakistan, HIV prevalence is increasing among IDUs. In Karachi, one study found a dramatic increase in HIV prevalence among IDUs, from under 1 percent in 2004 to 26 percent in 2005. The Ministry of Health (MOH) found that 48 percent of IDUs in Karachi and 82 percent in Lahore had used nonsterile syringes in the week before a 2004 survey. A study among IDUs in Karachi and Rawalpindi found only about half knew HIV could be transmitted through unclean needles. IDUs and sex workers are Burma's most-at-risk populations (MARPs), with 43 percent and 32 percent, respectively, found to be HIV-positive in 2005, according to UNAIDS. However, the epidemic is showing signs of a decline, with HIV prevalence among pregnant women at antenatal clinics dropping from 2.2 percent in 2000 to 1.5 percent in 2006.

The Central Asian Republics of Kazakhstan, Kyrgyzstan, Tajikistan, Turkmenistan, and Uzbekistan still have relatively low HIV prevalence. Nonetheless, recent sharp increases in the number of new infections, high prevalence in vulnerable populations, and the position of these countries at the crossroads of the drug-trafficking routes between Asia and Europe suggest that they are highly vulnerable to a rapid acceleration of the epidemic. Among the five Republics, Uzbekistan is experiencing the most dynamic epidemic. The number of new infections increased exponentially between 1999 and 2003, from 28 to 1,836, primarily due to injecting drug use combined with commercial sex. Since then, the annual number of newly reported HIV infections has grown at a slower pace, reaching 2,205 in 2006. In Kazakhstan, newly registered HIV cases increased from 699 in 2004 to 1,745 in 2006. The increase may be attributed in part to expanded HIV testing rather than to an increasing rate of infection. HIV has made less dramatic inroads in Kyrgyzstan, Turkmenistan, and Tajikistan, but prevalence among IDUs is a growing concern. Each of these countries reported fewer than 200 new HIV cases in 2005. In Tajikistan, the epidemic has grown among IDUs, and total annual newly diagnosed HIV infections increased from 7 in 2000 to 204 in 2006. In Kyrgyzstan, newly diagnosed HIV infections increased from 1 6 in 2000 to 244 in 2006.

HIV/AIDS is also a highly stigmatized illness in Asia because of its association with sexual and drug use behaviors. Often, it affects those considered to be outside the mainstream of society, including MSM, IDUs, and sex workers. The level and type of discrimination varies from country to country. For example, in Vietnam half of the men would keep their family member's HIV status a secret, whereas only 21 percent of men in the Philippines would do so. Failure to address stigma can deter individuals from getting tested, further perpetuating the epidemic. Addressing stigma and discrimination will require a comprehensive multisectoral response that includes changing social and cultural beliefs and behaviors and modifying policies at the government, employer, and educational levels.

HIV co-infection with tuberculosis (TB) is a major concern for the Asia region. According to the World Health Organization, the Asia region has the highest rates of TB in the world, and 11 out of the world's 22 high-TB-burden countries are Asian countries. HIV suppresses the immune system, which makes a person more susceptible to contracting TB. TB is also one of the main causes of death among HIV-positive persons. In Asia, more than 2 million people with TB are co-infected with HIV. The HIV prevalence rate among incident TB cases in the Asia region ranges from 0 percent in Bangladesh and TimorLeste to 10 percent in Cambodia. Kazakhstan and Uzbekistan have the majority (65 and 27 percent, respectively) of co- infected cases in the Central Asian region.

ECONOMIC AND SOCIAL IMPACT OF HIV/AIDS IN THE ASIA REGION

Illness, disability, and death associated with the HIV/AIDS epidemic have harmful social and economic effects. The majority of people who have the disease are between the ages of 15 and 49, and often the under-30 age group is the most affected. In **Kyrgyzstan**, for instance, 54.6 percent of all identified HIV/AIDS cases have occurred among 15- to 29-year-olds. This changes a population's demographic structure and poses a challenge to the systems in supporting dependent populations such as children and the elderly.

The economic and social effects of HIV/AIDS are felt from the family level, where families experience the death and incapacity of loved ones, to providers who must cope with the burden of caring for the sick and dying. The International Labor Organization found in 2003 that the average monthly expenditures for families of people living with HIV/AIDS in New Delhi exceeded income, in part because of the costs of medications. Food security is threatened by the effects on food production and the reduced ability of households to afford a nutritious diet. School enrollments decline, and the payoffs of investments in education are undercut by high death rates among young adults.

The economic costs of addressing HIV/AIDS and its effects, both in the health sector and other economic sectors, divert resources from other important needs and from investments critical to economic development. UNAIDS estimated in 2002 that providing antiretroviral therapy (ART) to all those in need in the Mekong subregion alone would cost $250 million in 2007. The costs also divert resources from other public health issues. For instance, a 2003 United Nations Development Program (UNDP) assessment in Vietnam suggested that mounting a comprehensive response to HIV/AIDS could absorb nearly 5 percent of public health spending by 2007. In many cases, the impact of the epidemic on families, communities, and countries has feedback effects that influence the epidemic's future course. For example, poverty and the breakdown of social and economic systems impair community systems that could help stem the spread of infection. The World Bank estimates that, if unchecked, the growing epidemic in Central Asia would slow economic growth over the next decade by 20 percent in Uzbekistan and by 10 percent in Kazakhstan and Kyrgyzstan.

Poor women in the Asia region are particularly vulnerable to HIV/AIDS. Poor economic circumstances can limit a woman's mobility and force her to stay in situations where her physical and emotional well-being are at risk. Dispossessing women of land and other means of production at home and the lack of formal skills to participate in economic activities can lead women to travel to urban areas in search of work. If they are unable to find a job, some are forced into commercial sex work or other vulnerable situations that can increase their risk of contracting HIV. Human trafficking is increasing in all the Mekong subregion countries. Women trafficked into sex work are particularly vulnerable to HIV. They tend to work in lower-class, often underground, brothels where they may be forced to service several clients each day. They often have no power to insist on condom use, even if they understand the risk of HIV/AIDS and other sexually transmitted infections (STIs).

Finally, HIV/AIDS has orphaned many children who are now raised by extended family members. In Thailand's Chiang Mai province, for instance, a large proportion of children who have lost one or both parents to AIDS are being cared for by grandparents and other extended family members, according to a 2004 study cited by UNAIDS. As parents die, the effects on children cannot be overstated. Many children orphaned by HIV/AIDS lose their childhood and are forced by circumstances to become income and food producers or caregivers for sick family members. They suffer their own increased health problems related to increased poverty and inadequate nutrition, housing, clothing, and basic care and affection.

NATIONAL/REGIONAL RESPONSE

The urgency of the issue and the ease with which HIV/AIDS crosses borders is prompting the Asia region and subregions to pursue a coordinated response to the epidemic. In 2007, the South Asia region held an intercountry consultation on the prevention of HIV among IDUs. Multisector country teams participated from Afghanistan, Bangladesh, Burma, India, Nepal, Pakistan, and Vietnam. Actions were identified to scale up HIV prevention among IDUs. At the Central Asian Conference on HIV/AIDS in 2001, the governments of Kazakhstan, Kyrgyzstan, Tajikistan, and Uzbekistan approved a declaration committing their countries to scaling up national responses and to the following priority actions: HIV prevention among IDUs; prevention and care interventions for STIs; the development and expansion of health promotion programs for young people, especially those most vulnerable; and the creation of a supportive legal, policy, and cultural environment. Although Turkmenistan did not send a representative to the conference, the government endorsed the declaration.

Most countries in the region have HIV/AIDS programs and policies. Although institutional capacity and financial resources are limited, many countries are making progress in responding to the epidemic. However, challenges remain, and stigma and discrimination persist.

The following are examples of the status of United States Agency for International Development (USAID)-assisted countries' HIV/AIDS policies and programs:

- India has taken an aggressive stance toward HIV/AIDS since 2004, implementing the third phase of its National AIDS Control Programme, designed to reverse the spread of HIV/AIDS by 2012. The country is mobilizing its response by using prevention, care, support, and treatment; increasing funding for HIV/AIDS activities; and establishing the National AIDS Council.
- Cambodia's National Strategic Plan for a Comprehensive and Multisectoral Response to HIV/AIDS, 2001–2005 concentrates on changing individual behaviors and the socioeconomic, legal, and political environment. The National Strategic Plan for 2006–2010 builds upon this approach and calls for expanded HIV sentinel surveillance and behavioral surveillance systems.
- Thailand reinvigorated its HIV/AIDS prevention and control efforts in 2006. Thailand's HIV/AIDS activities include conducting a public education campaign, improving STI treatment, discouraging men from visiting sex workers, promoting condom use, and requiring sex workers to receive monthly STI tests and carry records of their test results.
- Vietnam's National Strategic Plan on HIV/AIDS Prevention, 2004–2010 provides the framework for a national response to the epidemic, calling for mobilization of government-, party-, and community-level organizations across multiple sectors.
- Pakistan's Medium Term Development Framework, 2005–2010 includes among its goals the halving of HIV/AIDS prevalence in MARPs and pregnant women. The new National Strategic Framework, 2007–201 1 broadens the scope of HIV/AIDS control efforts established by the Framework for 2002–2006 by including women, children, and young adults in prevention efforts.
- The Government of Kazakhstan is implementing its National AIDS Program for 2006–2010. The program has three objectives: stabilize HIV prevalence by preventing the spread of infection from MARPs to the general population; reduce the incidence of HIV among MARPs; and ensure that at least 80 percent of HIV-infected individuals are covered by medical and social programs.
- Kyrgyzstan stands out in the region for its innovative and early response, establishing the Multisectoral Coordination Committee on HIV/AIDS, Tuberculosis, and Malaria in 1997. The government has actively sought assistance from nongovernmental organizations (NGOs) and international organizations for its prevention plan, which includes among its objectives: reducing the number of HIV-infected people, slowing the spread of HIV, and decreasing the incidence of STIs.
- Tajikistan's National Strategic Plan for 2007–2010 includes the following elements: a multisectoral approach; confidentiality in testing; integration of HIV/AIDS prevention and care into other health programs; establishment of a national coordinating mechanism; and dissemination of information among youth and other at-risk populations.
- In 2005, Turkmenistan approved the National Program on HIV/AIDS/STI Prevention for 2005–2010. The Program's goals include preventing HIV and other STIs among at-risk populations; preventing transmission of HIV and STIs through blood transfusions, by sexual intercourse, and from mother to child; and reducing morbidity from STIs.

- Uzbekistan's Strategic Program on Responding to HIV/AIDS for 2003–2006 led to the implementation of preventive services for at-risk populations and the integration of HIV-related lessons into educational programming; completion of second-generation HIV epidemiological surveillance; the launch of ART programs; and the establishment of a network for HIV-infected individuals and centers providing health services for youth. The Strategic Program on HIV/AIDS for 2007–2010 builds upon these successes while addressing major barriers to HIV prevention, treatment, care, and support, such as low demand for condoms and stigma and discrimination.

Businesses have a stake in responding to the epidemic that affects their workforce and can reduce the markets for their goods. As a result, the private sector is becoming more involved in HIV prevention efforts as shown through the following examples from India and China. Reliance Industries Limited, India's largest private sector company, established a medical center to treat TB and AIDS. Company physicians and local NGOs reached 300,000 people through prevention, testing, counseling, and ART. In China, UNDP launched an HIV awareness campaign with EPIN Technologies, a leading player in the country's new media industry. The campaign reached millions of passengers on board trains through education clips with basic facts about HIV/AIDS and the need to treat those living with HIV/AIDS with tolerance.

The Global Fund to Fight AIDS, Tuberculosis and Malaria has approved grants to most Asian countries to implement HIV/AIDS responses. The U.S. Government provides one-third of the Global Fund's contributions.

USAID REGIONAL SUPPORT IN ASIA

USAID programs in Asia are implemented in partnership with the President's Emergency Plan for AIDS Relief. The Emergency Plan is the largest commitment ever by any nation for an international health initiative dedicated to a single disease. To date, the U.S. has committed $1 8.8 billion to the fight against the global HIV/AIDS pandemic, exceeding its original commitment of $15 billion over five years.

Reauthorized on July 30, 2008, the U.S. is continuing its commitment to global AIDS in the amount of $39 billion for HIV/AIDS bilateral programs and contributions to the Global Fund to Fight AIDS, Tuberculosis and Malaria. Working in partnership with host nations, the initiative will support antiretroviral treatment for at least 3 million people, prevention of 12 million new HIV infections, and care and support for 12 million people, including 5 million orphans and vulnerable children (OVC).

In Asia, USAID work with PEPFAR places special emphasis on the focus countries of Vietnam, as well as Cambodia and India. In addition, HIV/AIDS programs are also implemented in a number of other countries, including Bangladesh, Burma, China, East Timor, Indonesia, Kazakhstan, Kyrgyzstan, Laos, Nepal, Pakistan, Papua New Guinea, the Philippines, Tajikistan, Turkmenistan, Thailand, and Uzbekistan.

Examples of USAID assistance include the following activities and interventions:

- USAID implemented a program in Bangladesh to assist local NGOs working with vulnerable groups to educate people on HIV risk reduction, improve knowledge about and treatment for other STIs, minimize contextual and policy-related constraints concerning HIV/AIDS, increase linkages between prevention and care, and improve monitoring and evaluation of HIV prevention programs.
- In Cambodia, USAID assisted with referrals for OVC and HIV-positive women to receive care and treatment from other agencies.
- In India, 23,000 individuals received ART in 2006.
- In Vietnam, 202,500 pregnant women in 2006 received mother-to-child transmission services.
- USAID transferred state-of-the-art national surveillance capacity to Indonesia's Central Bureau of Statistics and Ministry of Health; provided training for staff and equipment to perform quality diagnostic services and treatment to 91 HIV counseling and testing sites and 66 STI clinics in nine provinces; and initiated HIV/AIDS counseling and testing at TB sites in DKI Jakarta and Central Java.
- In China, USAID-supported programs increased levels of condom use among MARPs in hot-spot locations.
- In Kazakhstan, USAID supported the MOH's implementation in 2006 of a pilot program for prevention of mother-tochild HIV transmission. By the end of the year, reported data indicated that the rate of HIV prophylactic treatment for mothers increased from 44 to 83 percent and that treatment for newborns increased from 21 to 76 percent.
- In Tajikistan, USAID supported the enrollment of 115 drug users in a USAID-funded drug-free treatment and rehabilitation program.
- In Turkmenistan, USAID provided technical assistance to the government to develop the National Tuberculosis Prevention and Control Program and the HIV/AIDS Prevention Program for 2005–2010 and, in conjunction with the Centers for Disease Control and Prevention, signed a Memorandum of Understanding with Turkmenistan to implement a blood safety program. A Memorandum of Understanding has been signed between USAID and the Ministry of Health and Medical Industry to establish a youth center in Ashgabat.
- In Uzbekistan, USAID conducted HIV prevention outreach broadcasts on 18 mass media features and reached 1,500 migrants and about 3,000 children with messages on HIV prevention and drug use through interpersonal communication.
- With USAID funding, CDC has been implementing sentinel surveillance in four Central Asian countries since 2002. In Kazakhstan, sentinel surveillance is now implemented nationwide with funding from the government. CDC only provides technical assistance and training. In Kyrgyzstan, Tajikistan, and Uzbekistan, CDC leveraged resources from a World Bank-funded project to expand the model to more pilot sites. Laboratories receive technical assistance in establishing internal and external quality controls.

Recent USAID successes in the Central Asian Republics include awarding more than 50 grants to NGOs and government organizations and developing protocols to establish treatment readiness, drug-free treatment, and rehabilitation centers for drug users in

Uzbekistan, Tajikistan, and Kyrgyzstan through the Drug Demand Reduction Program (DDRP). The centers have already reached around 3,000 drug users. Since 2003, DDRP has provided vocation and drug demand reduction education to 460 vulnerable women; reached 1,500 rural-to-urban migrants through its drug demand reduction education and referral system; and trained more than 3,500 professionals.

IMPORTANT LINKS

USAID HIV/AIDS Web site for Asia: http://www.usaid.gov/our_work/global_health
For more information, see USAID's HIV/AIDS Web site: http://www.usaid.gov/our_work/global_health

In: Global HIV/AIDS Threat and the U.S. Response
Editor: David R. Carmody

ISBN: 978-1-61324-568-2
© 2011 Nova Science Publishers, Inc.

Chapter 8

HIV/AIDS HEALTH PROFILE - LATIN AMERICA AND THE CARIBBEAN

United States Agency for International Development

OVERALL HIV TRENDS

Most HIV epidemics in the Latin America and Caribbean (LAC) region appear to be stable, although in some Caribbean countries, they appear to be in decline. In 2007, about 69,000 people in LAC countries died of AIDS, and 117,000 were newly infected (UNAIDS, November 2007). The number of people living with HIV/AIDS (PLWHA) in LAC is estimated at 1 .8 million (UNAIDS, November 2007). Two-thirds of PLWHA reside in the four largest countries – Argentina, Brazil, Colombia, and Mexico – although the Caribbean and Central American subregions have higher prevalence rates, with countries such as Haiti and Belize having rates in 2005 as high as 3.8 and 2.5 percent, respectively (see figure below). With its large population, Brazil accounts for about one-third of PLWHA in the region. The epidemics in LAC are being fueled by varying combinations of unsafe sex (both between men and between men and women) and injecting drug use, but it is important to note that HIV/AIDS transmission patterns have moved increasingly from marginalized groups toward the general population (UNAIDS, December 2006). HIV prevalence among sex workers is relatively high in Central America and the Caribbean, especially in the Dominican Republic, Jamaica, Guyana, Honduras, Guatemala, and El Salvador (UNAIDS, November 2007). Unprotected sex between men is an important factor in Bolivia, Chile, Ecuador, Peru, El Salvador, Guatemala, Honduras, Mexico, Nicaragua, and Panama (UNAIDS, November 2007). Prevalence among men who have sex with men (MSM) may well be underestimated throughout the region because of stigma, the often hidden nature of this behavior, the fact that some MSM also have sex with women, and the small numbers of people engaging in risky behaviors who actually know their status. Between 1986 and 2004, 27 percent of the HIV/AIDS cases in Argentina, Uruguay, Paraguay, and Chile were attributed to injecting drug use, and over the same time period in Brazil, 16 percent of cases were transmitted through injecting drug use (USAID, 2006). However, HIV prevalence in Brazil among injecting drug users (IDUs) is declining in some cities as a result of harm reduction programs, mortality among IDUs, and a change from injecting to inhaling drugs (UNAIDS and WHO, 2006). In Argentina and Uruguay, the epidemics are driven mainly by unprotected heterosexual intercourse (UNAIDS, November 2007).

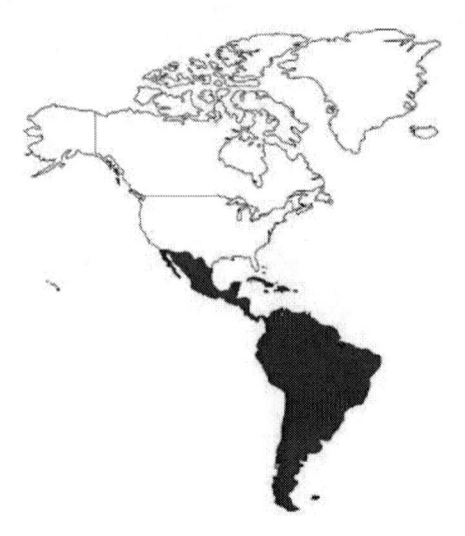

The figure on the previous page shows trends in HIV/AIDS prevalence in the LAC region between 2003 and 2005. In most countries, the prevalence rate showed little change or was in decline, although in a few it continued to rise. Increases were particularly notable in Peru, Belize, the Bahamas, and Suriname. Haiti remains one of the region's high-prevalence countries, with 3.8 percent of the adult population HIV-positive (UNAIDS, 2006) (although a more recent population-based survey suggests that the national HIV prevalence rate could be significantly lower).

The Caribbean's status as the second-highest HIV prevalence region in the world masks substantial differences in the extent and intensity of its epidemics. Two countries, Haiti and the Dominican Republic, have nearly three-quarters of all the infections in the Caribbean, but national HIV prevalence is high (between 1 and 3.8 percent) throughout the subregion (UNAIDS, December 2006, November 2007). New infections remain stable in the Dominican Republic. A sentinel surveillance study in 2006 reported that prevalence among commercial sex workers (CSWs) ranged from 2.4 to 6.5 percent and averaged 4.1 percent. In some sites, prevalence among CSWs is declining and equals that of pregnant women. In Haiti, HIV prevalence among pregnant women attending antenatal clinics declined from 5.9 percent in 1996 to 3.1 percent in 2004 (UNAIDS, November 2007). In 2006, sentinel surveillance results among pregnant women suggested a stabilization of HIV prevalence, and modeling of Haiti's epidemic suggests that the declining trends are due to mortality and an increase in protective behaviors. Behavioral surveys demonstrate a 20 percent decline in the mean number of sex partners between 1994 and 2000, while condom use increased among nonregular partners (UNAIDS, November 2007). However, localized trends suggest the need to protect against a resurgent epidemic. HIV prevalence among pregnant women in rural areas has not decreased, and only 16 percent of women and 3 1 percent of men in rural areas used a condom the last time they had casual sex (UNAIDS, December 2006). The epidemics in the Caribbean are fueled by multiple sexual partners, a thriving sex industry, and MSM. A 2005–2006 behavioral surveillance survey from six eastern Caribbean countries found that 3 1 to 46 percent of the surveyed population aged 15 to 24 had multiple sexual partners within the last 12 months. New infections among women are surpassing those among men. Young women in particular face considerably higher odds of becoming infected than young men (UNAIDS, 2005); their higher risk is exacerbated by cross-generational sex and the "sugar daddy" phenomenon (i.e., reliance of younger women on older men for material needs, often basic, in exchange for sex). In Haiti, new data from the Ministry of Public Health and Population show that in some areas, the prevalence rate of HIV infection among young women is twice that of young men.

The LAC region has made considerable progress in providing antiretroviral therapy (ART). According to the April 2007 WHO/UNAIDS/UNICEF progress report *Towards Universal Access,* the number of people receiving ART in LAC steadily increased from 210,000 in 2003 to 355,000 in 2007. There are considerable variations across countries, but the overall coverage of 72 percent appears to be approaching universal access.

HIV/AIDS-tuberculosis (TB) co-infection is a problem in many parts of LAC. In certain countries and provinces where TB incidence is high, there is a need to coordinate HIV/AIDS and TB services. In some areas, people dying from HIV/AIDS are succumbing to TB. In the states of Rio de Janeiro and Sao Paulo, Brazil, HIV-TB co-infection runs as high as 25 percent in the major cities. The Dominican Republic has one of the highest TB incidence rates in the Americas, at 9 1 cases per 100,000 population. Although data on co-infection are limited, it is estimated that 6 to 11 percent of TB patients in the Dominican Republic are also infected with HIV. Therefore, the Dominican Republic represents a case where there is the potential for a burgeoning epidemic of TB along with HIV.

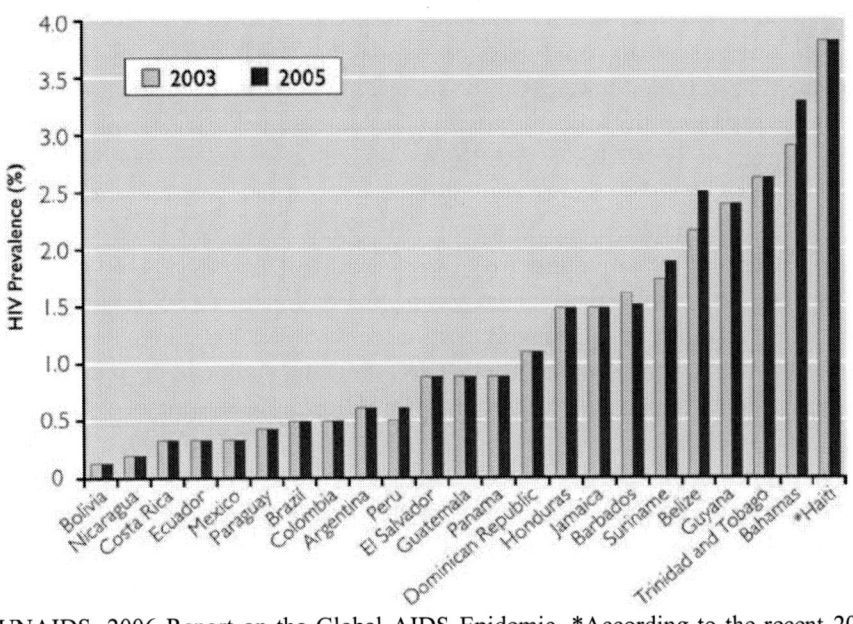

Source: UNAIDS. 2006 Report on the Global AIDS Epidemic. *According to the recent 2005–2006 Survey on Mortality, Morbidity, and Utilization of Services, Haiti's national prevalence rate may be as low as 2.2 percent.

Trends in HIV Prevalence, 2003–2005.

ECONOMIC AND SOCIAL IMPACT OF HIV/AIDS IN LATIN AMERICA AND THE CARIBBEAN

Illness, disability, and death associated with HIV/AIDS affect populations at multiple levels and in multiple ways. The vast majority of people who have the disease are between the ages of 15 and 49, and often, the under-30 age group is the most affected. This has an impact on the most economically active part of a population, resulting in possible changes in the demographic structure that pose challenges to support systems for dependent populations such as children and the elderly.

HIV/AIDS epidemics cut the supply of labor and threaten the livelihoods of many workers. According to a 2004 report from the International Labour Organization (ILO), from 1990 to 2010, Haiti could lose more than 10 percent of its labor force to HIV/AIDS if the availability of ART is inadequate. The loss of skilled and experienced workers causes productivity to fall and business costs to increase, and tax revenues, market demand, and investment are also undermined. Studies suggest, however, that a company's investment in prevention, medical care for opportunistic infections such as TB, and treatment of sexually transmitted infections (STIs) reduces personnel turnover rates and labor costs. Preliminary research shows that the cost of providing treatment and care to keep employees in the workforce is often less than the cost of replacing workers lost to HIV/AIDS, even for small businesses. Volkswagen in Brazil reports that its AIDS care program has reduced costs to the company from between $1,500 to $2,000 per affected employee per month to $300 (*Action Against AIDS in the Workplace*, UNAIDS, August 2005). VARIG, the largest airline company in Latin America, realized that the nature of its work placed the company's employees in situations that could lead to risk-taking behavior. In 1986, the company introduced an AIDS program to respond to the health and social needs of its employees and "fulfill a social responsibility role by contributing to national and international efforts to control the impact of HIV/AIDS." VARIG's 2003 budget for prevention activities and medication was approximately $5 per employee per year. Employees and their families have free access to voluntary counseling and testing (VCT) and ART. VARIG extends its program beyond the workplace by providing free cargo handling for selected drugs that are not available in Brazil and sponsoring annual campaigns on World AIDS Day. Also in Brazil, Nestlé (the world's largest food company with more than 254,000 employees worldwide) is seeing the results of its long-standing HIV/AIDS program. Its focus on prevention through behavior change has resulted in a reduction of more than 50 percent of workers reporting high-risk behavior. Other key components of Nestlé's policy include nondiscrimination against PLWHA, confidentiality, and disclosure. Benefits include VCT, care, support, and treatment for employees, spouses, and their children. Business coalitions to fight HIV/AIDS are engaged in similar efforts in Mexico, Jamaica, and other Caribbean countries.

The economic and social effects of HIV/AIDS are felt from the family level, where families experience the death and incapacity of loved ones and providers must cope with the burden of caring for the sick and dying, to businesses, schools, hospitals, and other institutions that suffer the loss of valuable personnel and declines in productivity. In many cases, the impact of the epidemics on families, communities, and countries has feedback effects that influence the epidemics' future course; for example, poverty and the breakdown of social and economic systems impair community systems that could help stem the spread of infection. Food security is threatened by the effects on food production and the reduced ability of households to afford a nutritious diet. School enrollments decline, and the payoffs of investments in education are undercut by high death rates among young adults.

The economic costs of addressing HIV/AIDS and its effects, both in the health sector and other economic sectors, divert resources from other important needs and from investments critical to economic development. A study by CAREC and the University of the West Indies Health Economic Unit, for example, estimated that Jamaica's gross domestic product could be 6.4 percent lower by 2005 due to HIV/AIDS. According to ILO's model, income in eight LAC countries would have grown by 0.5 percent more per year without the HIV/AIDS epidemics (2004). A study sponsored by the World Economic Forum, Harvard School of Public Health, and UNAIDS *Business and HIV/AIDS: Commitment and Action: A Global Review of the Business Response to HIV/AIDS (2004–2005)*, found that, overall, 1 6 percent of the nearly 9,000 business leaders surveyed from 104 countries judged HIV/AIDS a serious business threat. Moreover, 35 percent of respondents in Latin America and 67 percent in the Caribbean expected some impact of HIV/AIDS on their companies in the next five years.

Finally, HIV/AIDS has orphaned many children who are now raised by grandparents, live in orphanages, or live in households headed by other children. As parents die, the effects on children cannot be overstated. Many children orphaned by HIV/AIDS lose their childhood and are forced by circumstances to become producers of income and food or caregivers for sick family members. They often drop out of school and suffer their own increased health problems related to increased poverty and inadequate nutrition, housing, clothing, and basic care and affection.

PARTNERING FOR SUCCESS: USAID AND THE U.S. PRESIDENT'S EMERGENCY PLAN FOR AIDS RELIEF

The United States Agency for International Development (USAID) programs in LAC are implemented in partnership with the U.S. President's Emergency Plan for AIDS Relief (Emergency Plan/PEPFAR). The Emergency Plan is the largest commitment ever by any nation for an international health initiative dedicated to a single disease. To date, the U.S. has committed $1 8.8 billion to the fight against the global HIV/AIDS pandemic, exceeding its original commitment of $15 billion over five years.

Reauthorized on July 30, 2008, the U.S. is continuing its commitment to global AIDS in the amount of $39 billion for HIV/AIDS bilateral programs and contributions to the Global Fund to Fight AIDS, Tuberculosis and Malaria. Working in partnership with host nations, the initiative will support antiretroviral treatment for at least 3 million people, prevention of 12 million new HIV infections, and care and support for 12 million people, including 5 million orphans and vulnerable children.

The Emergency Plan encompasses all U.S. Government (USG) international HIV/AIDS activities, including those implemented by USAID. Under the Emergency Plan in LAC, USAID's staff of foreign service officers, trained physicians, epidemiologists, and public health advisers work with host governments, nongovernmental organizations (NGOs), and the private sector to provide training, technical assistance, and supplies – including pharmaceuticals – to prevent and reduce the transmission of HIV/AIDS and provide care and treatment to PLWHA. In fiscal year 2008, USAID will continue efforts to prevent the spread of HIV/AIDS using several interventions:

- The ABC approach to preventing sexual transmission of HIV – Abstinence, Be faithful, correct and consistent use of Condoms
- Prevention of mother-to-child HIV transmission (PMTCT)
- VCT services
- Injection safety and ensuring the safety of blood supplies
- Provision of therapy for concurrent illnesses and opportunistic infections, as well as palliative care
- Nutritional therapy
- Support for OVC
- Strengthening the supply chain for critical commodities
- Strategic information including public health evaluations and health and behavioral studies

A proposal has been made to extend the Emergency Plan for another five years and $50 billion dollars. There appears to be bipartisan support for this effort, and it is expected that the expanded PEPFAR program will continue through 201 3.

USAID is uniquely positioned to support multisectoral responses to HIV/AIDS that address the widespread impact of HIV/AIDS outside the health sector. In particular, USAID is supporting cross-sector programs in areas such as agriculture, education, democracy, and trade that link to HIV/AIDS and mutually support the objective of reducing the impact of the pandemic on nations, communities, families, and individuals. Under the Emergency Plan, USAID also supports a number of international partnerships; provides monetary and technical support to the Global Fund to Fight AIDS, Tuberculosis and Malaria and its grantees in LAC; and works with local coordinating committees of the Global Fund to improve implementation of its programs and their complement to USG programs. Finally, USAID supports targeted research, development, and dissemination of new technologies and new packaging and distribution mechanisms for antiretroviral drugs.

USAID Support in Latin America and the Caribbean

USAID plays a lead role in coordinating the activities of several USG agencies in the region in support of PEPFAR, including the U.S. Centers for Disease Control and Prevention (CDC), the Peace Corps, the U.S. Department of Labor, and the U.S. Department of Defense. In LAC, USAID and PEPFAR place special emphasis on two focus countries – Guyana and Haiti. In addition, HIV/AIDS programs are also implemented in a number of other countries, including Belize, Bolivia, Brazil, the Dominican Republic, El Salvador, Guatemala, Honduras, Jamaica, Mexico, Nicaragua, Peru, and Panama. In addition, USAID's Caribbean Regional Program covers Trinidad and Tobago, Suriname, St. Kitts and Nevis, St. Lucia, St. Vincent and the Grenadines, Grenada, Antigua and Barbuda, Dominica, and Barbados. In the Caribbean, USAID is also an active member of the Pan Caribbean Partnership on HIV/AIDS, providing support on both a bilateral and regional basis, including increasing the capacity of

NGOs and community organizations to deliver HIV/AIDS prevention and care programs and improving governments' capacity to implement an effective response.

Examples of recent USAID assistance include the following activities and interventions:

- In collaboration with the Health Resources and Services Administration and CDC, USAID has provided substantial technical and financial assistance toward the establishment of six training centers, known as CHART (Caribbean HIV/AIDS Regional Training), in Jamaica, the Bahamas, Barbados, Haiti (2), and Trinidad and Tobago, providing training to health professionals in more than 30 countries in the region. In 2006, 69 1 HIV/AIDS service providers were trained; they in turn provided services in 3 15 VCT sites and 46 ART clinics where more than 7,000 HIV-positive patients received treatment.
- In Bolivia, USAID strengthened the national HIV/AIDS prevention program by conducting a research study on hard-toreach groups to develop prevention messages; developed a manual for HIV/AIDS VCT; and opened VCT sites in five NGO health service delivery centers with high-risk populations. To expand access to VCT, especially for at-risk populations, 90 health providers received training in VCT in 2006.
- In Brazil, USAID is supporting prevention projects developed by Brazilian NGOs to improve the quality of life for PLWHA. Activities are geared toward focusing on overall quality of life issues that have been identified as high priorities by PLWHA, such as treatment adherence, nutritional literacy, income generation, job skills training, and improving linkages to other social movements. USAID in collaboration with CDC supported the completion of a TB-HIV co-morbidity study.
- In the Dominican Republic, USAID reached more than 250,000 adolescents and youth with abstinence and being faithful messages through the annual youth and adolescent song contest; reached 117,000 people with testing and counseling services; supported PMTCT services in 82 facilities for almost 72,000 women and their babies; provided direct support to six outpatient clinics; supported treatment for 11,552 HIV-positive patients; and supported 7,669 OVC through 18 community- and home-based care programs for children and families affected by HIV/AIDS.
- In Guyana, USAID supported prevention programs emphasizing abstinence and being faithful for 33,900 people annually and reached 28,300 people with counseling and testing services. PMTCT services have reached nearly national coverage, and USAID has significantly strengthened a joint partner procurement and supply chain system.
- In Haiti, USAID supported prevention programs emphasizing abstinence and being faithful for 345,700 people; counseling and testing for 128,600 people; palliative care and support for 38,700 people; and program assistance for 20,000 OVC.
- In Mexico, USAID supported the launch of a successful HIV/AIDS business council (known as CONAES) dedicated to the elimination of job-based discrimination. CONAES has 30 member companies from a diverse range of Mexican and multilateral businesses. Since 2004, CONAES has had a direct impact on 150,000 Mexican workers and an indirect impact on an estimated 560,000 family members. Private companies contributed more than $400,000 of their own resources, and in

December 2006, CONAES became completely self-sustaining through member contributions.

- In Peru, USAID conducted a number of activities aimed at reducing stigma and discrimination (S&D), including training health professionals; developing and testing a monitoring system to include S&D as a criterion for quality of care; successfully promoting the inclusion of HIV/AIDS-related S&D on the agenda of the Peruvian ombudsman; and producing guidelines to decrease S&D in families of PLWHA. USAID reached 65,200 individuals through a communication program to prevent HIV/AIDS; trained 187 health professionals in VCT; and completed two baseline surveys on knowledge of STIs and HIV/AIDS and safer sexual behaviors among MSM, sex workers, and PLWHA.
- In Suriname, USAID launched a media campaign that significantly increased HIV/AIDS counseling and testing between December 2005 and August 2006. Client satisfaction has improved and staff workload has decreased since the implementation of same-visit testing and results.

IMPORTANT LINKS AND CONTACTS

Latin America and Caribbean Bureau/RSD-PHN, #5.9.101
USAID
1300 Pennsylvania Avenue, N.W.
Washington, D.C. 20523-5900
Phone: 202-712-4964
Fax: 202-216-3262
E-mail: lstewart@usaid.gov
Web site: http://www.usaid.gov/locations/latinamericacaribbean/issues

For more information, see USAID HIV/AIDS Web site http://www.usaid.gov/ourwork/globalhealth/aids

Caribbean Regional Program Web site http://www.usaid.gov/ourwork/globalhealth/aids/Countries/lac/caribbeanregion.html

Central America Regional Program Web site http://www.usaid.gov/ourwork/globalhealth/aids/Countries/lac/caregion.html

In: Global HIV/AIDS Threat and the U.S. Response
Editor: David R. Carmody

ISBN: 978-1-61324-568-2
© 2011 Nova Science Publishers, Inc.

Chapter 9

HIV/AIDS HEALTH PROFILE - EUROPE AND EURASIA REGION

United States Agency for International Development

OVERALL HIV TRENDS

Eastern Europe and Central Asia is the only region where HIV prevalence clearly continues to increase, with an estimated 130,000 new infections in 2009 alone. In the same year, 1.4 million adults and children were living with HIV in Eastern Europe and Central Asia. From 2001 to 2008, there was a 66 percent increase in the total number of people living with HIV/AIDS (PLWHA); in comparison, prevalence in sub-Saharan Africa fell from 5.8 percent to 5.2 percent, and prevalence in Southeast Asia stabilized in the same period. Eastern Europe is also the only region where the annual number of HIV-related deaths continues to rise, increasing fourfold from 18,000 in 2001 to 76,000 in 2009.

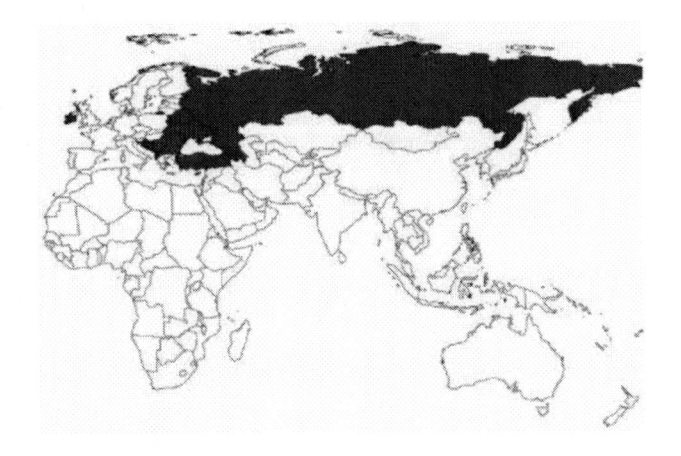

In Eastern Europe, injecting drug use continues to be the primary form of transmission, accounting for 57 percent of new HIV infections in 2007, according to the Joint United Nations Program on HIV/AIDS (UNAIDS). However, heterosexual transmission accounted for 42 percent in the same year, and the proportion of new infections through sexual transmission has been growing as the epidemic moves from injecting drug users (IDUs) to their partners. Increases in prevalence among women are linked to the epidemic through IDUs. An estimated 35 percent of women living with HIV acquired the virus through injecting drugs, and 50 percent of HIV-positive women contracted the disease by having sex with IDUs. In Ukraine, the hardest hit country in the region, sexual transmission of HIV outpaced transmission via injecting drug use for the first time in 2008, although HIV prevalence still seems focused among IDUs and their partners. In the same year, a study in Russia found that having sex with an IDU increased the risk of acquiring HIV by 3.6 times compared to having sex with a non-IDU. With 66 percent of IDUs in Russia having had sex with noninjecting partners in the past year, there is a high risk of transmission to non-IDUs.

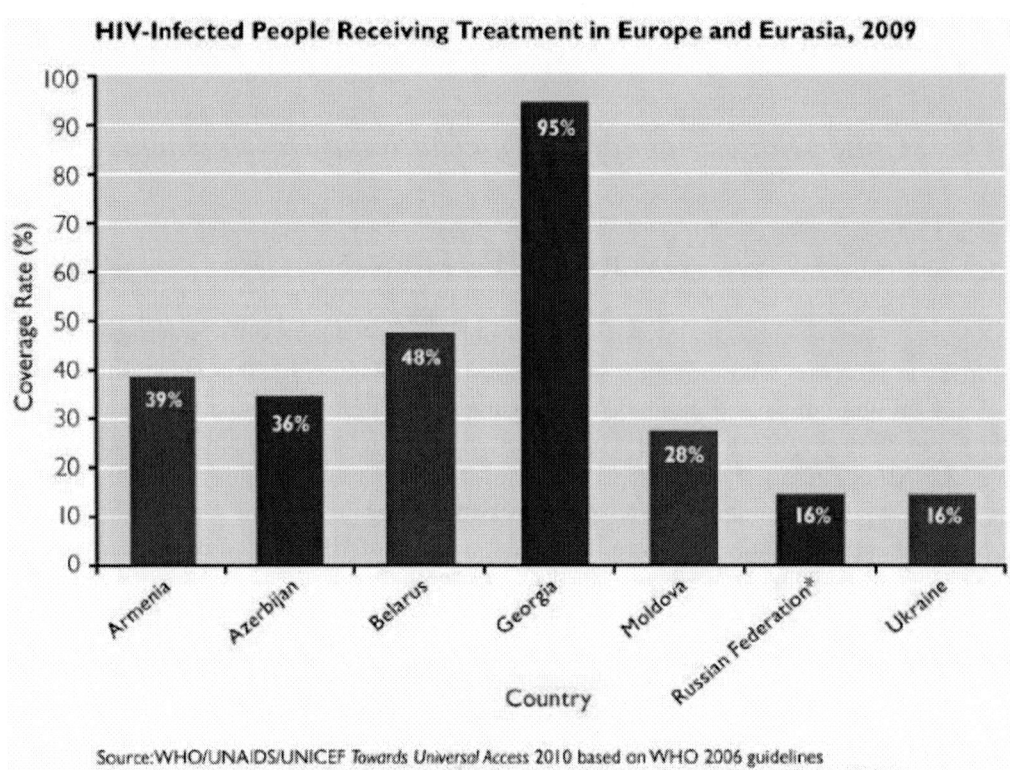

HIV-Infected People Receiving Treatment in Europe and Eurasia, 2009

Source: WHO/UNAIDS/UNICEF *Towards Universal Access* 2010 based on WHO 2006 guidelines
*Russian Federation data from WHO/UNAIDS/UNICEF *Towards Universal Access* 2008, data for end 2007

The severity of the HIV epidemic in the countries of Eastern Europe and Eurasia (E&E) varies widely, from concentrated epidemics in Ukraine and Russia to low-level epidemics in Armenia and Georgia. Ukraine has the highest HIV prevalence rate in the E&E region, with an estimated adult prevalence of 1.1 percent in 2009 and more than twice as many annual HIV diagnoses than in 2000. Russia and Ukraine together account for approximately 90 percent of all people newly reported to be living with HIV in the region, according to UNAIDS. Particularly high HIV prevalence has been found among drug users in both countries; studies in select regions and cities found prevalence between 39 and 50 percent in Ukraine and as high as 37 percent in Russia.

Sex workers are one most-at-risk population (MARP) in E&E, especially those who engage in transactional sex with IDUs. HIV prevalence rates among sex workers varied greatly between and within countries – as high as 20 percent in Irkutsk, Russia, in 2009, and from 14 to 31 percent in Ukraine. A 2006 study in St. Petersburg focusing on sex workers under 19 years of age found an HIV prevalence of 33 percent. Infection among IDUs and sex workers is often linked because these two high-risk populations overlap. Some sex workers inject drugs, while some IDUs do sex work to earn money for drugs. In Russia, at least 30 percent of sex workers were found to have injected drugs in the past, according to UNAIDS.

Men who have sex with men (MSM) comprise the third major MARP in the E&E region. Official estimates of HIV transmission and prevalence among MSM are thought to be grossly underestimated, according to UNAIDS. Moreover, the data that do exist for this population are limited because the stigmatization of MSM discourages men from accurately reporting their high-risk behaviors. In a 2009 study of 14 cities in Ukraine, prevalence among MSM was as high as 8.6 percent, more than five times the prevalence in the general population.

HIV Estimates in Europe and Eurasia Region[*]	
Armenia	
Total Population	3.0 million
Estimated Number of Adults and Children Living with HIV/AIDS	1,900
Adult HIV Prevalence	0.1%
Azerbaijan	
Total Population	8.3 million
Estimated Number of Adults and Children Living with HIV/AIDS	3,600
Adult HIV Prevalence	0.1%
HIV Prevalence Among IDUs (Baku, 2008)	10.3%
HIV Prevalence Among Female Sex Workers (Baku, 2008)	1.7%
HIV Prevalence Among MSM (Baku, 2008)	1.0%
Belarus	
Total Population	9.6 million
Estimated Number of Adults and Children Living with HIV/AIDS	17,000
Adult HIV Prevalence	0.3%
HIV Prevalence Among IDUs (Minsk, 2009)	13.7%
HIV Prevalence Among Female Sex Workers (Minsk, 2009)	6.4%
HIV Prevalence Among MSM (Minsk, 2009)	2.7%
Georgia	
Total Population	4.6 million
Estimated Number of Adults and Children Living with HIV/AIDS	3,500
Adult HIV Prevalence	0.1%
HIV Prevalence Among IDUs (Tbilisi, 2008)	2.2%
HIV Prevalence Among Female Sex Workers (Tbilisi, 2009)	2.0%
HIV Prevalence Among MSM (Tbilisi, 2007)	3.6%
Moldova	
Total Population	4.3 million
Estimated Number of Adults and Children Living with HIV/AIDS	12,000
Adult HIV Prevalence	0.4%
HIV Prevalence Among CSWs (2009)	6.1%

Continued

HIV Estimates in Europe and Eurasia Region[*]	
Russia	
Total Population	139.4 million
Estimated Number of Adults and Children Living with HIV/AIDS	980,000
Adult HIV Prevalence	1.0%
HIV Prevalence Among IDUs (National, 2009)	15.6%
HIV Prevalence Among IDUs (St. Petersburg, 2009)	61.2%
HIV Prevalence Among MSM (2009)	8.3%
HIV Prevalence Among Commercial Sex Workers (2009)	4.5%
Ukraine	
Total Population	45.4 million
Estimated Number of Adults and Children Living with HIV/AIDS	350,000
Adult HIV Prevalence	1.1%
HIV Prevalence Among IDUs (30 territories, 2008–2009)	22.9%
HIV Prevalence Among MSM (14 cities, 2009)	8.6%
HIV Prevalence Among Sex Workers (25 territories, 2008–2009)	13.2%

[*] HIV data are not available for Albania and Kosovo.
Total Population: U.S. Census Bureau
Number of PLWHA and HIV Prevalence: UNAIDS
HIV Prevalence among MARPS: UNAIDS, UNGASS Country Progress reports

Treatment coverage remains low in all E&E countries except Georgia, as illustrated in the graph on the first page. Access to antiretroviral therapy (ART) is expanding, however; from 2003 to 2007, the number of people receiving ART increased from 15,000 to 54,000. The concentration of HIV in MARPs and other hard-to-reach populations is a challenge in increasing ART coverage, as these populations often have limited access to health services. In 2009, the World Health Organization (WHO) issued revised recommendations about when adults, adolescents, and pregnant women should initiate ART. WHO now recommends ART be initiated when the CD4 white blood cell count reaches or drops below 350 cells/mm^3, rather than the 2006 recommendation of 200 cells/mm^3. This change immediately increased the number of PLWHA who are eligible for and in need of treatment, and WHO anticipates it will reduce HIV-related morbidity, mortality, and hospitalization in the long term.

Increases in the number of PLWHA receiving treatment are having profound effects on HIV-related mortality in many countries in the E&E region due to prolonged life and reduced annual deaths from HIV/AIDS. Prevention of motherto-child transmission (PMTCT) coverage in the region was the highest in the world. In Ukraine, WHO estimates between 76 and 95 percent of HIV-positive pregnant women received antiretroviral drugs for PMTCT in 2009.

Ukraine has the highest estimated adult HIV prevalence in the E&E region, at 1.1 percent. In 2009, sexual transmission accounted for almost 44 percent of new infections. Despite this, the epidemic continues to be concentrated in IDUs and other MARPs. For example, transmission by injecting drug use accounted for 36 percent of new infections in 2009. In 2008 and 2009, HIV prevalence among IDUs in 30 territories averaged 22.9 percent, and prevalence as high as 55.2 percent was recorded among IDUs in the city of Mykolaiv. Limited knowledge of HIV fuels the spread of the virus: Fewer than half of men and women in the country have a comprehensive understanding of how to reduce the risk of infection, according to the 2007 Ukraine Demographic and Health Survey. Lack of opioid substitution therapy and limited needle exchange programs for IDUs, as well as stigma and discrimination against IDUs and PLWHA, fuel the continued spread of the virus in the IDU population.

With an estimated adult HIV prevalence of 1 percent, Russia has the second highest HIV prevalence in the region. By 2009, an estimated 980,000 people in Russia were living with HIV. The prevalence in the country remained low through 1996, when 1,515 new cases were reported in connection with an outbreak among IDUs, and started to increase dramatically after 2003. Transmission through injecting drug use accounted for 62 percent of new infections in 2009, but, as in Ukraine, the proportion of new HIV infections due to injection drug use has fallen, and sexual transmission is on the rise. In 2007, more than one-third of new cases were attributed to sexual transmission, although data suggest the epidemic is still concentrated among IDU populations and their partners.

Adult HIV prevalence in Georgia has slowly increased over the past decade to 0.1 percent in 2009; in the same year, the country was home to approximately 1,200 PLWHA. The epidemic continues to be driven by injecting drug use, which accounts for 60 percent of new infections, but heterosexual transmission has become more common in recent years (34 percent of new cases). The majority of PLWHA are men, with three HIV-positive men for every HIV-positive woman. Despite having a low overall prevalence, widespread injecting drug use puts the country at risk of a broader epidemic.

In Armenia, prevalence remains low; 823 cases of HIV were officially diagnosed as of December 2009, and UNAIDS estimates 1,900 people are currently living with HIV/AIDS. The number of new cases of HIV has been on the rise in recent years, with the highest number of cases (149) of any year diagnosed in 2009. While marked increases in the number of new infections reported may be skewed by increases in testing and scale-up of laboratory capacity, the increases are still a reason for concern. Heterosexual sex accounts for 50 percent of cases, and injection drug use accounted for an additional 41 percent; most infections among men are attributed to injecting drug use, while 98 percent of infections in women are through sexual transmission.

In 2009, Belarus had 1,500 new HIV infections, according to UNAIDS, and the annual rate of new infections has held steady since 2003. UNAIDS indicated the estimated adult HIV prevalence tripled, from 0.1 percent in 2001 to 0.3 percent in 2009. The epidemic is concentrated among IDUs; in the city of Zlobin, prevalence rates as high as 52 percent were reported among IDUs in 2006.

The number of newly diagnosed HIV infections in Moldova has increased almost fourfold since 2001, although the estimated adult prevalence has remained fixed at 0.4 percent over the past decade due to HIV-related mortality. While transmission through injecting drug use was the dominant cause of infection in the late 1990s and early 2000s, heterosexual sex has been the primary mode of transmission since 2004. Nearly all pregnant women are tested for HIV, and prevalence among this group was approximately 0.29 percent in 2009. Recent surveillance data from 2009 found a prevalence of 6.1 percent among commercial sex workers (CSWs), markedly higher than among the general population.

Low HIV prevalence in some E&E countries, such as Albania, Kosovo, and Azerbaijan, must be considered with caution due to the risk of continued spread of the virus. Albania is a very low prevalence country, with more than 90 percent of new infections transmitted through sexual contact. The majority of PLWHA are in the capital city of Tirana. Kosovo is home to

43 known cases of HIV, and the majority of these cases are among males aged 30 to 39; however, the actual number is estimated to be much higher. Based on limited available data, the country is experiencing a low-level epidemic. Azerbaijan is another low-prevalence country, with an estimated 0.1 percent prevalence in the adult population, although the country experienced a 16.2-percent increase in the rate of newly diagnosed HIV infections from 2005 to 2006.

While the U.S. Agency for International Development's (USAID's) E&E Bureau no longer runs programs in the Baltics, HIV continues to be a major challenge in the area. The rate of new HIV diagnoses has declined since 2003, although the HIV incidence rate in Estonia – the highest in WHO's European region – is 504.2 to 626.3 per 1 million population; the country's estimated adult prevalence in 2007 (1.3 percent) was one of the highest in the E&E region. The history of HIV in Estonia is one of the most pointed examples of how the virus can spread quickly through use of shared injecting drug equipment. A limited number of cases had been detected in the country a decade ago, but within a few years the majority of IDUs surveyed (up to 72 percent in some surveys) were HIV positive, according to UNAIDS. By 2007, 62.5 percent of IDUs in the capital city of Tallinn were living with HIV.

HIV-tuberculosis (TB) co-infection complicates the care and treatment of both diseases. HIV weakens the body's ability to fight TB, the most common AIDS-associated disease in the region. Estimated TB incidence varies throughout the region, according to WHO. In Russia, estimated TB incidence was 106 new TB cases per 100,000 population in 2009; in Ukraine, incidence was 101 per 100,000 population. In Russia, 4 percent of people with TB are co- infected with HIV; in Ukraine, 11 percent of people with TB also have HIV, the highest co-infection rate in the region.

ECONOMIC AND SOCIAL IMPACT OF HIV/AIDS IN EUROPE AND EURASIA

The cost of addressing HIV can divert resources from investments critical to economic development on a national level, and from meeting day-to-day needs on a family level. HIV infection can drain a family's resources due to increased medical expenses. It can also leave a house with one or no income-earning adult. As has been demonstrated in other countries, the impact of the epidemic on families and communities influences the epidemic's future course. HIV-related morbidity and mortality can change a population's demographic and economic structure when younger, normally productive members of society are unable to work or die from complications related to HIV. Some parents who die from complications associated with HIV/AIDS leave behind young children who are also HIV positive. Such children often do not receive medical care and suffer social isolation and discrimination. Although the prevalence of HIV currently remains low in most countries of the region, the continued growth and spread of the epidemic will create ongoing challenges to development.

While the economic effects of HIV/AIDS remain limited in the E&E region, their impact is beginning to be felt in countries with larger epidemics, including Russia and Ukraine. In Ukraine, a 2006 World Bank study estimated a 1 to 6 percent reduction in gross domestic product (GDP) from 2004 to 2014 as a consequence of the growing HIV epidemic. The same World Bank study predicted a 1 to 2 percent reduction in the labor force due to the epidemic;

it also estimated that the 20 to 34 age group would account for three-quarters of all new HIV infections by 2014, if HIV/AIDS programming continues at 2006 levels. In Russia, a separate non-intervention scenario from the World Bank estimated the country's GDP could decline by as much as 10.7 percent as a result of the epidemic. The costs of HIV/AIDS care and treatment also divert resources from other important health investments.

HIV prevention among mobile populations is becoming increasingly important to controlling the epidemic, as many migrant workers travel from Central Asia to Russia for work. When migrant workers are away from their families for extended periods of time, they tend to engage in risky behavior, which puts them and their respective partners at home at greater risk of contracting HIV. Immigrants often lack access to health services, including HIV prevention and treatment, compounding the risk of spreading the epidemic.

Stigma and discrimination toward PLWHA, especially toward those who belong to marginalized groups, can contribute to further spread of the virus when members of these groups are reluctant to access health services; MSM and IDUs living with HIV often face stigma both for their positive status and for belonging to stigmatized groups. Stigma against PLWHA encompasses a range of behaviors, including gossip and verbal abuse, violence and physical abuse, and discrimination when seeking employment.

When HIV-positive individuals are reticent about disclosing their HIV status, they cannot receive the proper care and treatment or be counseled on methods of preventing the spread of HIV. Negative attitudes and behaviors often deter PLWHA from seeking services at health facilities due to fear of stigmatization and discrimination by health workers. A small study by USAID reported discriminatory attitudes toward PLWHA hindered health workers' ability to provide high-quality care. A survey across three *oblasts* in Ukraine found that while most health workers received HIV/AIDS-related training, half thought it was insufficient, and nearly one-third thought HIV-positive patients should be treated in isolation in order to prevent the spread of infection to other patients and staff.

The United Nations Development Program found that the majority of people living in the E&E region fear the discrimination associated with being HIV positive more than they fear the actual health effects and complications of infection. PLWHA who disclose their status often have difficulty finding employment or face discrimination at work, relegating them to informal employment or low-skill, low-wage positions. For PLWHA who are also MSM, IDUs – or both – the chances of finding employment are reduced even further.

NATIONAL/REGIONAL RESPONSE

The transition away from communism throughout the former Soviet Bloc countries resulted in systemic restructuring throughout the E&E region. During the 1990s, budget shortfalls during the rebuilding process led to compromised public health systems in many countries, creating challenges in the early response to HIV. More recently, the Commonwealth of Independent States (CIS)[1] developed a Coordinating Council on HIV through which member states cooperate on scaling up access to ART under WHO's former "3 by 5" initiative and other AIDS-related initiatives. In 2006, the first Eastern European and Central Asian AIDS Conference was held in Moscow, with all countries in the region coming together to discuss urgent issues and examine strategies to overcome challenges. The participants emphasized evidence-based, nondiscriminatory care and the use of civil society groups, the private sector, and other stakeholders as partners in the implementation of a response. Despite this promising rhetoric, there continues to be many challenges to adequately address and combat the HIV epidemic throughout the E&E region.

Country responses to the epidemic vary throughout the region.

- Ukraine has actively worked to stop the spread of HIV since the early 1990s. In 2005, the national response was reinvigorated with the establishment of the National Coordination Council on HIV/AIDS. Additional policies and programs were developed to expand access to treatment, care, and family planning services for PLWHA. The country has also introduced opioid substitution therapy for IDUs and harm reduction programs to address the population most affected by the epidemic; many of these services are supported by grants from the Global Fund to Fight AIDS, Tuberculosis and Malaria. Despite expanded programs, a UNAIDS evaluation found sex workers and MSM remain largely hidden and unreached populations.

- In Russia, the Government recognizes HIV infection as one of the major threats to national security and the health of the nation, with the disease spreading with increasing frequency from MARPs to the general population. Federal funding for the response to HIV has grown rapidly since 2005, and the Government has made a number of commitments to address the HIV/AIDS epidemic. Government programs focus primarily on treatment of AIDS rather than prevention, care, and support, although they have a widely implemented PMTCT program. In 2009, approximately 9,380 pregnant women received antiretroviral drugs for PMTCT, according to UNAIDS.

- Georgia has mainstreamed HIV prevention and control activities since 1994, prioritizing voluntary counseling and testing, reaching MARPs, providing free PMTCT services, building capacity, and raising local awareness through media campaigns. As of 2008, the Government also supported opioid substitution therapy as a response to the widespread use of injected heroin; a limited Government-sponsored detoxification program started in the same year.

- In 2003, Albania created a network of strategic partners to respond to HIV, and the current response to the epidemic is guided by the National Strategic Plan for 2008–2014. A new law passed in 2008 addresses the most critical legal aspects of HIV/AIDS, including discrimination, the right to keep one's job, informed consent, confidentiality, and the establishment of safe places for care and treatment.

- Armenia passed landmark human rights amendments to the law on HIV prevention in March 2009. The U.S. Government (USG) provides nearly 30 percent of the Global Fund's total contributions worldwide. From 2003 to 2010, the Global Fund has approved grants to countries in Eastern Europe and Central Asia totaling nearly $763 million (the majority of which are grants for activities in Russia and Ukraine). These grants have targeted high-risk groups, including IDUs, CSWs, youth, street children, prisoners, uniformed personnel, and migrants. Programs support a broad range of accessible services to reduce these groups' vulnerability to infection as well as referral to treatment and care services for people living with HIV. A number of grants are for integrated HIV-TB services. However, as grants come to an end across the region, it will be important to work with governments to ensure they are taking on the responsibility for these key programs and funding them.

USAID REGIONAL SUPPORT

USAID's HIV/AIDS programs in the E&E region are implemented as part of the U.S. President's Emergency Plan for AIDS Relief (PEPFAR). Launched in 2003, PEPFAR is the USG initiative to support partner nations around the world in responding to HIV/AIDS. Through PEPFAR, the USG has committed approximately $32 billion to bilateral HIV/AIDS programs and the Global Fund through fiscal year 2010. PEPFAR is the cornerstone of the President's Global Health Initiative (GHI), which supports partner countries in improving and expanding access to health services. Building on the successes of PEPFAR, GHI supports partner countries in improving health outcomes through strengthened health systems, with a particular focus on improving the health of women, newborns, and children.

USAID programs in the region prioritize prevention activities to decrease HIV infections and help contain the epidemic in the E&E region. Currently, USAID provides both country and regional support for prevention, care, and support programs. The Agency also provides technical assistance to a range of countries to help them develop HIV/AIDS programming and obtain funding from the Global Fund. USAID programming focuses on reaching high-risk populations by providing assistance to local governments and organizations to improve access to effective and high-quality services. Programs include prevention of sexual and biomedical transmission; care for those affected and infected with HIV, including orphans and vulnerable children; improving access to treatment; support to create political will to combat the epidemic; and support of policies addressing stigma and discrimination of PLWHA.

HIV/AIDS activities in 2009 included the continuation of the regional medication-assisted therapy (MAT) policy project. The MAT project is intended to provide information and resources for 10 countries: Albania, Armenia, Azerbaijan, Georgia, Kazakhstan, Kyrgyzstan, Russia, Tajikistan, Ukraine, and Uzbekistan. The goal of the project is to create tools that will assist local advocates and policymakers in building public policy foundations that support the implementation and expansion of evidence-informed drug dependence services, particularly opioid substitution maintenance therapy.

Throughout the E&E region, country programs had significant achievements in 2009. In Georgia, for example, the USG is one of the few providers of HIV prevention services for MARPs and supports organizational capacity building throughout the country. In Russia, programs reached more than 86,000 individuals with HIV prevention activities in 2009; they also expanded coverage to 6,400 IDUs and approximately 12,000 CSWs and their partners in the same year. A partnership with a Russian organization, Transatlantic Partners Against AIDS, helped mobilize high-level official, business, and mass media partners to address the epidemic through policy research, information, analysis, and workplace initiatives. An additional partnership with the American International Health Alliance provided training in basic HIV skills and knowledge to more than 1,100 health care workers, teachers, and social workers as part of an effort to strengthen the HIV/AIDS treatment and care service delivery system.

In 2009, USAID technical support facilitated the preparation and adoption of 11 policy and regulatory documents on HIV issues by the Government of Ukraine. These issues included the National AIDS Law; voluntary counseling and testing for MARPs; methadone-based treatment for HIV-infected IDUs; HIV/AIDS drug and commodity procurement; and support for vulnerable children. In addition, training 75 civil society representatives in advocacy enabled PLWHA, nongovernmental HIV service organizations, and MARP representatives to work more efficiently with policymakers.

Important Links

USAID's HIV/AIDS Web site for Europe and Eurasia: http://www.usaid.gov/locations/europeeurasia/health

For more information, see USAID's HIV/AIDS Web site:_http://www.usaid.gov/ourwork/globalhealth/aids.

End Notes

[1] The following countries make up the CIS: Armenia, Azerbaijan, Belarus, Georgia, Kazakhstan, Kyrgyzstan, Moldova, Russia, Tajikistan, Turkmenistan, Ukraine, and Uzbekistan.

CHAPTER SOURCES

The following chapters have been previously published:

Chapter 1 – This is an edited reformatted and augmented version of a Congressional Research Service publication, report R41645, dated February 22, 2011.

Chapter 2 – This is an edited reformatted and augmented version of a United States President's Emergency Plan for AIDS Relief publication, report *Five-Year Strategy*.

Chapter 3 - This is an edited reformatted and augmented version of a United States President's Emergency Plan for AIDS Relief publication, report *Five-Year Strategy, Annex: PEPFAR and Prevention, Care, and Treatment*.

Chapter 4 - This is an edited reformatted and augmented version of a United States President's Emergency Plan for AIDS Relief publication, report *Five-Year Strategy, Annex: PEPFAR and the Global Context of HIV*.

Chapter 5 – This is an edited reformatted and augmented version of a United State Government Accountability Office publication, report GAO-10-836, dated September 2010.

Chapter 6 – This is an edited reformatted and augmented version of a United States Agency International Development publication, report *HIV/AIDS Health Profile, Africa Region*.

Chapter 7 – This is an edited reformatted and augmented version of a United States Agency International Development publication, report *HIV/AIDS Health Profile,Asia Region*.

Chapter 8 – This is an edited reformatted and augmented version of a United States Agency International Development publication, report *HIV/AIDS Health Profile, Latin America and the Caribbean*.

Chapter 9 – This is an edited reformatted and augmented version of a United States Agency International Development publication, report *HIV/AIDS Health Profile, Europe and Eurasia Region*.

INDEX

E